Sex, Work and Professionalism

Sex, Work and Professionalism examines what happens when professional concern is defined in terms of sex. Based on original fieldwork with outreach workers in HIV prevention it addresses issues of professionalism, emotion work and boundaries, integrating empirical insights with sociological theory.

In most professional relationships sex is not defined as part of the relationship, in fact it is explicitly excluded in guidelines and codes of ethics. HIV prevention outreach workers work in sexual environments with a sexually defined target group and are often employed on the basis of their sexuality. They have to learn how to balance their work and professional lives, overcoming conflicts such as:

- professional role versus community role
- sexual skills versus sexual boundaries
- personal experiences versus professional understanding
- professional identity versus worldviews.

Many of the questions being raised in this book about the meaning of professionalism, the pain and pleasure in emotion work and the management of boundaries between home, sex and work are being asked more generally by workers in a range of organisations. *Sex, Work and Professionalism* argues for a new understanding of professionalism more appropriate to the human services.

Katie Deverell works in new product development for Unilever Research. She is also Visiting Research Fellow at South Bank University. She has previously worked in HIV prevention and evaluation.

Social Aspects of AIDS

Series Editor: Peter Aggleton
Institute of Education, University of London

AIDS is not simply a concern for scientists, doctors and medical researchers, it has important social dimensions as well. These include individual, cultural and media responses to the epidemic, stigmatisation and discrimination, counselling, care and health promotion. This series of books brings together work from many disciplines including psychology, sociology, cultural and media studies, anthropology, education and history. The titles will be of interest to the general reader, those involved in education and social research, and scientific researchers who want to examine the social aspects of AIDS.

Recent titles include:

Imagine Hope
Simon Watney

AIDS in Europe: New Challenges for the Social Sciences
Edited by Jean-Paul Moatti, Yves Souteyrand, Annick Prieur, Theo Sandfort and Peter Aggleton

Dying to Care? Work, Stress and Burnout in HIV/AIDS
David Miller

Mental Health and HIV Infection
Edited by José Catalán

The Dutch Response to HIV: Pragmatism and Consensus
Edited by Theo Sandfort

Families and Communities Responding to AIDS
Edited by Peter Aggleton, Graham Hart and Peter Davies

Men Who Sell Sex: International Perspectives on Male Prostitution and AIDS
Edited by Peter Aggleton

Sexual Behaviour and HIV/AIDS in Europe: Comparisons of National Surveys
Edited by Michel Hubert, Nathalie Bajos and Theo Sandfort

Drug Injecting and HIV Infection: Global Dimensions and Local Responses
Edited by Gerry Stimson, Don C. Des Jarlais and Andrew Ball

AIDS as a Gender Issue
Edited by Lorraine Sherr, Catherine Hankins and Lydia Bennett

AIDS: Activism and Alliances
Edited by Peter Aggleton, Peter Davies and Graham Hart

Sexual Interactions and HIV Risk: New Conceptual Perspectives in European Research
Edited by Luc Van Campenhoudt, Mitchell Cohen, Gustavo Guizzardi and Dominique Hausser

Bisexualities and AIDS: International Perspectives
Edited by Peter Aggleton

Social Aspects of AIDS

Series Editor: Peter Aggleton
Institute of Education, University of London

Editorial Advisory Board:

Sex, Work and Professionalism
Working in HIV/AIDS

Katie Deverell

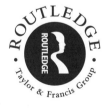

London and New York

First published 2001
by Routledge
11 New Fetter Lane, London EC4P 4EE

Simultaneously published in the USA and Canada
by Routledge
29 West 35th Street, New York, NY 10001

Routledge is an imprint of the Taylor & Francis Group

Typeset in Times New Roman by Bookcraft Ltd, Stroud, Gloucestershire
Printed and bound in Great Britain by Biddles Ltd, Guildford and Kings Lynn

British Library Cataloguing in Publication Data
A catalogue record for this book is available from the British Library

Library of Congress Cataloging in Publication Data
Deverell, Katie.
  Sex, work, and professionalism: working in HIV/AIDS / Katie Deverell.
    p. cm. – (Social aspects of AIDS)
  Includes bibliographical references and index.
  1. AIDS (Disease) – Prevention – Social aspects.   2. Health
  education – Social aspects.   3. Public health personnel – Attitudes.
  4. Public health personnel – Sexual behavior.   I. Title.   II. Series.

RA643.8 .D48 2001
362.1'969792–dc21
                                                    2001020491

ISBN 0–415–23320–8 (hbk)
ISBN 0–415–23321–6 (pbk)

Contents

Figures

Acknowledgements

There are many people who helped in different ways to produce this book and I am thankful to them all. The most important contributors were the HIV prevention workers I interviewed and worked with. Without their interest and involvement the production of this book would not have been possible. I found the fieldwork immensely enjoyable and hope that I have done justice to the views I collected.

Peter Aggleton played an invaluable role as a supportive and constructive editor. His advice and suggestions were not only motivating but also helped sharpen and enrich the text. Mike Savage, Angie Hart, Alan Prout and Ursula Sharma all took time to read parts of the manuscript. The book has greatly benefited from the different viewpoints they expressed. In addition, many people provided valued friendship, peer support and time to discuss ideas. The following deserve special mention: Will Anderson; Jason Annetts; Tina Bird; John Britt; Martin Calleja; Penni Charteress; Marie-Elena Costa Sa; Tom Doyle; Kevin Eisenstadt; Philip Gatter; Robin Gorna; Mike Hartley; Ford Hickson; Kea Horvers; Ben Kernighan; Jane Mezzone; David Miller; David O'Donnell; Andrew Prentice; Mark Reedman; Andrew Ridley; J. Russell; Jamie Taylor; Ian Warwick; members of the Southbank University Sexuality reading group and the trustees and workers from The LADS Project.

Finally, thanks to the Deverells and Whites for their continual support and encouragement. In particular to Alex, who helped in numerous practical and emotional ways, and, importantly, encouraged me to develop some boundaries of my own by tempting me away from writing!

I would like to thank the following for their kind permission to reproduce extracts from copyright works: *Annual Review of Sociology* for Freidson, E. (1984) 'The changing nature of professional control' *Annual Review of Sociology* 10: 1–20; Cambridge University Press for Andrews, M. (1991) *Lifetimes of Commitment: Aging, Politics, Psychology*; Bailey, J. (2000) 'Some Meanings of "the private" in sociological thought' *Sociology*, 34(3): 381–401; Craib, I. (1995) 'Some comments on the sociology of the emotions' *Sociology*, February, 29(1):151–9; Tonkiss, F. and Passey, A. (1999) 'Trust, confidence and voluntary organisations: between values and institutions' *Sociology* 33(2): 57–274; Harper Collins Publishers for extracts from the *Collins English Dictionary* 1990; Macmillan Press Ltd for Halford, S., Savage, M. and Witz, A. (1997) *Gender,*

Careers and Organisations, Current Developments in Banking, Nursing and Local Government; Routledge Ltd for Cavendish, R. (1982) *Women on the Line*; Sage Publications Ltd for Lyon, K. (1993) 'Why study roles and relationships?', in J. Walmsley, J. Reynolds, P. Shakespeare and R. Woolfe (eds) *Health Welfare and Practice: Reflecting on Roles and Relationships*; Macdonald, K. (1995) *The Sociology of the Professions*; Pringle, R. (1989) 'Bureaucracy, rationality and sexuality: the case of secretaries', in J. Hearn, D.L. Sheppard, P. Tancred-Sheriff and G. Burrell (eds) *The Sexuality of Organization*; Sheppard, D.L. (1989) 'Organizations, power and sexuality: the image and self-image of women managers', in J. Hearn, D.L. Sheppard, P. Tancred-Sheriff and G. Burrell (eds) *The Sexuality of Organization*; J. Walmsley, J. Reynolds, P. Shakespeare and R. Woolfe (eds) *Health Welfare and Practice: Reflecting on Roles and Relationships*; Williams, J. (1993) 'What is a profession? Experience versus expertise', in J. Walmsley, J. Reynolds, P. Shakespeare and R. Woolfe (eds) *Health Welfare and Practice: Reflecting on Roles and Relationships*.

Series editor's preface

HIV and AIDS pose a major challenge to public health all over the world. Even in the richer countries of Europe, North America and Asia-Pacific, health systems have often been slow to respond. While initially, relatively few health care workers wanted to become involved in HIV/AIDS-related work, with time there has been a growth of involvement. New ways of working and new occupational categories have come into existence. Among these is direct face-to-face work with vulnerable and heavily affected communities.

Prior to the advent of HIV/AIDS, relatively little health promotion work took place with marginal groups such as sex workers, people who inject drugs and homosexually active men. Either their existence was officially denied, or their needs were seen as somehow peripheral to more mainstream forms of health service provision. The epidemic has changed all that and it is increasingly recognised that work with especially vulnerable communities brings benefits, not only for the individuals concerned, but also for wider society. Outreach work, as it is often known, has become one of the mainstays of HIV prevention activity.

But who are the workers involved, and why do they commit themselves to work in stressful and sometimes dangerous conditions? What skills are needed to talk with strangers about intimate and sometimes risky sexual practices? And what are the consequences of this kind of work for professional and personal life? These are just some of the issues explored in this book. Its author, Katie Deverell, spent several years conducting in-depth research among community-based workers carrying out safer sex education among gay and bisexual men.

Her account offers a candid insight into the lives and practices of outreach workers – the barriers that have to be built between work and personal life, the complications that can ensue when clients want things to go a little too far, and the strategies used to legitimate this all important set of activities. *Sex, Work and Professionalism* offers a behind-the-scenes account of a little understood aspect of HIV prevention work. It raises important questions about the relationship between work and family life, professionalisation and the professions, and the role that insiders can play in health promotion work.

Peter Aggleton, London, June 2001

Introduction

My interest in the area of professionalism and boundaries initially developed from experience working first as a full time volunteer with the Terrence Higgins Trust (THT) in London, and later as a research assistant interviewing young people about sex. Working for the THT in the late 1980s had a profound influence on my life; although the work was often hectic, stressful and challenging it was a place where people were tremendously open, particularly about sex and sexuality, and where colleagues took great note of each other's well being. As one of my first jobs, this gave me a skewed idea of what working life was often like. Moving back to a university after working at THT seemed terribly sterile. However, discussions about sex and sexuality continued here as I was working on a funded project investigating how young people negotiate sexual encounters. For my fellow research assistant and I, such discussions were not only vital to the progress of the research they were also important personally, as we both felt changed by our work.

One thing that struck me when undertaking this sex-related research was the response to it from others in the department. Our work seemed to be treated as a bit of a joke. Talking to people about sex all day was seen as an easy, trivial job. Furthermore, some male colleagues seemed to find the research titillating and would wander into our office and casually attempt to read our interview transcripts, or suggest we sell tapes of the interviews to pornographic magazines. On the other hand we were constantly being told that: 'Nobody will tell you the truth', 'You won't get people to talk about sex'. These comments bore little resemblance to my experience of the interviews, in which people seemed to appreciate the chance to talk to someone openly and recount experiences they felt unable to tell a friend or family member. As the work progressed, I began to experience a widening gulf between the way I thought and talked about sex and sexuality, and the way a lot of other people did. It was not that I lacked a sense of humour about it – this was essential! Perhaps my interests just changed, or maybe it was no longer exciting, novel or naughty to discuss it?

Undertaking sex and HIV-related research also had an impact on my social life. For example, I often ended up giving impromptu HIV testing and safer sex advice sessions at parties. This seems similar to some doctors' experiences of being permanently 'on call'. In some ways this situation was useful, providing opportunities to reflect on ideas from the research. However, at times it made me feel isolated; I felt I had too academic a view of sex and sexuality. I seemed to spend all my time thinking and talking about it, while others actually did it. It was also wearing that telling people about my work often seemed to arouse sexual interest, or led to unwanted expectations of intimacy on my part. This was something noted by a medical friend who, as a consequence of discussing sex in the context of HIV with a male psychologist at a social function, received a card from him asking her to contact him if 'She ever wanted to talk about sex again'. She felt it was very hard to discern whether he was being flirtatious or just discussing work.

In 1990, I began work as the evaluation fieldworker for a community development initiative concerning the safer sex/HIV needs of men who have sex with men (Prout and Deverell 1995). I was intrigued to discover that the gay and bisexual male project workers interviewed were experiencing similar feelings to those I had found in the past. These included the ambiguity of personal–professional boundaries, challenges to identity and sexuality, the need to discuss with co-workers feelings about sex and sexuality, and their work being treated as a joke by others. It seemed that these issues were not just personal but related to the nature of the work itself. I therefore decided to carry out a specific study to explore the experiences of those in HIV-related work.

This book is the outcome of a qualitative research study addressing issues of sex, work and professionalism through the experiences of HIV prevention outreach workers. The focus on this occupation was chosen as it brings into sharp relief the ways in which sex, sexuality and work are linked. These workers have a professional concern defined in terms of sex and sexuality, work in sexual environments with a sexually defined target group, and are often employed on the basis of their own sexuality. For this reason, sex, sexuality and work are not seen to be separate and outreach workers do not experience a neat separation between their public and private lives. However, to gain funds, credibility and to avoid burnout, workers continually strive to manage the impact of their personal feelings on the work they do, and to separate their work and personal lives.

The study focused on gay and bisexual male workers who were working with gay, bisexual and other men who have sex with men. These workers reported a number of tensions created by having personal and work lives whose boundaries are blurred. These included having a specific (professional) role but being part of the community worked in; the need to use sexual skills to make contact with service users while maintaining sexual boundaries; and managing the extent to which personal experience is used within work. One of the ways in which HIV prevention outreach workers tried to balance these tensions was by developing 'professional' codes of conduct to guide their behaviour. Although not seeing themselves as a profession, rhetoric of 'professionalism' amongst this group was strong and clearly guided behaviour within and outside of work. Through in-depth exploration of their experiences, this book illuminates how understandings of appropriate professional behaviour guide practice on an everyday level, even for those in occupations not traditionally classed as professions.

In the past, most sociological work on professions has focused on defining which occupations count as true professions, or on processes of professionalisation. The focus in this book is quite different, looking at professionalism in terms of every-day practice to show how ideas of professionalism guide micro-level boundary-making behaviour. In this way, I highlight how professionalism can be seen as an identity rather than a set of job attributes. This focus on micro-level practices of professionalism and boundary making aims to show how outreach workers' day to day behaviour is influenced by funding systems, organisational structures, under-standings of sexuality, ideas about professionalism and the history of HIV preven-tion. Through addressing the links between these macro and micro experiences, the book demonstrates how tensions can occur where a worker's identity as a pro-fessional may conflict with his or her community attachment.

While the making of boundaries within work, and between work and other parts of people's lives has not been discussed in detail in many other occupations, many of the methods described by outreach workers are relatively common, e.g. having different places to socialise, changing clothes, putting aside time for leisure, and maintaining confidentiality. Indeed, interviewees often made spontaneous com-parisons between their roles and those of GPs, social workers and bankers. Perhaps the most usual comparison, however, was with counsellors and indeed much exist-ing literature related to boundaries has focused on the experiences of psychiatrists, counsellors and nurses. Although the book does not make detailed comparisons between different occupations, it does have practical application as a reflective aid in broader discussions of professional practice. The issues raised: the stress on life skills, identity, and personal experience rather than formal knowledge and qualifi-cations; how boundaries are made; the management of helping relationships; understandings of professionalism, and the role of trust in community based work all have broader relevance to those working in occupations such as social work, counselling, various voluntary sector organisations and community based health promotion. Indeed outreach workers' experiences help shed light on growing debates about the nature of professionalism and the relationship between work and other parts of life.

In Chapter one, I explore in more detail the theoretical background to the study by outlining four main themes: the critique of the distinction between public and private domains; new work on organisational sexuality; recent literature on profes-sional–client relationships; and continuing sociological debates about professions and professionalisation. The methods I used, and some of the methodological issues that arose, are discussed in Chapter two. Chapter three addresses the history and context of HIV prevention for gay men within Britain. It introduces important themes such as the association between gay men and HIV, the history of HIV pre-vention and tensions between statutory and community based work. The nature and place of outreach work are also discussed.

Having set the scene, Chapter four looks at why workers felt a need for bound-aries, by exploring how sex and sexuality form part of their work. The idea of sexual skills is developed here and I offer an outline of the various ways in which sexuality is used within work. Importantly, this is one of the first accounts to address issues of sex and work in the context of non-heterosexual relationships. Chapter five takes a contrasting perspective, considering how work impacted on people's personal social and sexual lives. Here, I look at the varied effects that undertaking HIV prevention had on interviewees and highlight the particular difficulties associated with living and working in the same elective community.

Having addressed why boundary making is important, but often difficult, the next two chapters look more closely at how boundaries were made within work, and between work and other parts of life. In Chapter six why such boundaries were felt to be important is explored in detail, along with how they were actively constructed through a process of negotiation with service users, managers and colleagues. The focus on an occupation that is developing ideas about appropriate professional conduct, and debating the purpose of its work, helps to emphasise the ways in which ideas about professionalism are negotiated and learnt. Chapter seven examines how notions of professionalism were used to guide workers' behaviour. By outlining how understandings of 'being professional' affected boundary making, this chapter argues that a more cultural understanding of being professional is needed. It also addresses the difficulties many gay men felt in describing themselves as 'professional' by examining the relationship between professionalism and sexual identity.

A concluding chapter discusses the findings in relation to wider theoretical debates about professionalism and boundary making. With the rise in service sector industries, issues of boundaries and professionalism are becoming more prominent as more workers have jobs that rely on the development of personal relationships. Indeed, with current organisational trends towards manufacturing and service cultures that operate on a 24-hour basis, a greater emphasis on individualised service, the use of skill-based teams and more informal, flatter organisations, issues of professionalism, work–life balance and personal boundaries are beginning to be discussed in many occupations. This book shows that despite the fairly unusual nature of their roles, elements of outreach workers' experiences have direct relevance to wider debates about the contemporary world of work.

Katie Deverell, Chester, 2000

Part 1

Orientations

1 Sex, work and professionalism

Theoretical issues

> The idea that 'work' can be clearly separated from 'home' retains both academic and popular appeal. In our research, this notion of *segmentation* was presented as both an organisational and an individual ideal. However, beneath this ideal it quickly becomes apparent that the boundaries between 'home' and 'work' are in fact blurred both in individual accounts and in organisational symbols, relationships and identities.
>
> (Halford *et al.* 1997:204–5)

Historically, it has been popular for sociologists to talk about the separation of home and work in terms of distinct public and private spheres. Sexuality, emotions and 'the personal' were seen to be separate from the rational, public world of work. Indeed, sex was more usually equated with leisure. In recent years this idea has been critiqued, particularly by feminist writers (Elshtain 1981; Haraway 1990; Stacey and Price 1981), and by new sociological studies of sex and sexuality at work. These and other writers have shown that despite the ideology of separate spheres, work and personal life are not clearly separate.

The public and the private

Within sociology there has been a tendency for sex to be regarded as something very separate from work; indeed at times almost its opposite (Finch 1983; Hearn and Parkin 1987). Weber argued that there was a split between the public world of rationality and efficiency and the private sphere of the emotional and personal life, and this notion has been vigorously taken up. Indeed, Bailey (2000) argues that 'Public and private are the common referents to deep and basic domains of social experience. They denote fundamental ordering categories in everyday life' (Bailey 2000:384).

The origins of the opposition between work and home can be traced to the rise of capitalism and the beginning of industrialisation, when it is argued the public sphere of work and the private domestic sphere became more sharply divided (Engels 1972). This led to a marked separation of roles and tasks between the world of home and leisure and the world of work. Within sociology, the dominance of the public–private distinction frequently led to sex and sexuality being seen as part of the 'personal sphere', belonging to the realm of home and family. Sexuality, the emotions and 'the personal' were something disruptive that must be kept out of the public world of work. For example, Gramsci wrote: 'the new type of man demanded by the rationalisation of production and work cannot be developed until the sexual instinct has been suitably regulated and until it too has been rationalised' (Forgacs 1988:282).

Parsons (1980) among others argued that efficiency at work depended on keeping personal considerations at bay, and Roy (1974) in an account of factory work suggests that sex is considered functionally and spatially inappropriate for industrial activity. Thus for the sake of production, sexuality and feelings were relegated to the personal world of home. For some writers, the home fulfilled a therapeutic and regulatory function: 'A wife and home siphon off the discontents which, if left untreated, would endanger his continued exploitation at work and threaten the very foundations of the production process' (Comer 1974:237–8).

Functionalist arguments such as these relied heavily on the idea of specific gender roles linked to the public–private distinction. Indeed, at times these arrangements seemed to be taken as 'natural'. However, the very fact that the world of work is seen as so vulnerable to contamination by sex and emotions points to the constructed nature of this dichotomy. If the public and private spheres were so firmly separate, there would be no cause for anxiety about sexuality and emotions disturbing the rational world of work.

The persistence of the public–private distinction, and its hold over the theoretical imagination, can be seen in the way that even those writers who recognise the socially constructed nature of this division still regard these separate spheres as complementary, and give specific qualities to each. For example, Fineman (1991) in an article on emotions and work seems to regard home as a place where one can be 'real', and suggests that family and home offer the usual complement to work in our society. More generally, there is a common sense notion that work and home are different, with home being seen, if not always experienced, as a haven from the cruel world of work (Lasch 1995; Saunders 1990). Cavendish (1982) for example, has argued that factory workers often see the family as making up for work, seeing it as an area of life beyond production, the market place and the arm of the state.

The idea of the complementarity of these two spheres has been critiqued by feminists who have argued that the public–private distinction has restricted and undervalued the role of women, who have become associated with the personal domestic sphere (Barrett and McIntosh 1982; Harris 1981). For example, those writing in what came to be termed the 'domestic labour debate' pointed out that housework has been undervalued because it has not been regarded as 'real' work (Glazer 1990; Oakley 1974). Because of this its contribution to economic production is not recognised, even though the feeding, clothing and emotional work done by many 'housewives' plays a crucial role. As Finch argues:

> In so far as wives do respond to these 'needs' created in work by providing what is regarded as an appropriate contrast – a comfortable, undemanding and

well-organised home – they can be seen as contributing their labour towards the production of a husband with a greater capacity for work.

(Finch 1983:367)

Gowler and Legge in the late seventies argued that: 'organisations tend to assume that (the) wives of their career committed employees will provide a flexible and supportive domestic environment' (1978:51), even though this work is unpaid, and often unrecognised. More recent work suggests that women frequently continue to play this support role even when they have careers of their own. Furthermore, women in heterosexual partnerships cannot separate home and work so easily as men because in most cases they still have greater responsibility for domestic tasks (Baxter and Western 1998; Halford *et al.* 1997; Sullivan 2000). The ideology of separate spheres can serve to obscure the links between home and work, leaving unrecognised much of the emotional and domestic labour necessary for a successful work life outside the home.[1]

One of the problems with portraying 'the home' as a complementary sphere to work is that such a comparison fails to recognise the many different ways in which households and domestic lives are organised. As this study focuses on the experiences of gay and bisexual men, it is significant that the existing literature focuses on (usually married) heterosexuals. Most gay men do not have wives and it is unclear what the relationship between home and work is for those gay men with long term live-in partners. In fact the idea of home as a complement to work fails to recognise the experiences of those living alone, unhappy at home, or who work at home. There is a need for a more detailed analysis of different domestic and partnership arrangements in order to understand how the relationship between home and work varies with regard to age, class, gender, sexuality and parental status.

A further problem with the construction of home and work as separate yet complementary is that it ignores the difference in influence which each sphere has. Far from being complementary, it could be argued that the demands of work often dominate home life. For example, an employee is more likely to take work home than bring their unfinished ironing to work (although this may change as some workplaces are now beginning to offer services such as dry cleaning on site). Work structures other parts of life and provides a framework into which other relationships must fit. Such a situation was highlighted by Cavendish, who when working (and studying) in a factory found that this left her time only for basic living:

> The struggle to keep going at such a basic physical level came as a shock to me; I hadn't anticipated what a strain the work would be and resented having to spend so much of my time out of work just recovering. Sleeping and eating became a much more central part of life.

(Cavendish 1982:123)

This is an experience many workers can relate too. Indeed Johnson (1983) has argued that the relationship between home and work is often full of tensions rather than being harmonious. He discusses how involvement in a career has implications for family life and how personal commitments may constrain career choices. For this reason, individuals may have to make important compromises between the different aspects of their lives.

The idea that we live our lives in two independent and completely separate spheres is obviously unrealistic and offers an idealised portrait of both 'the family' and home. Moreover, the use of binary oppositional categories between the public and private can mean that personal, emotional and sexual issues are often not dealt with at work. This is not just a theoretical issue but has practical implications. As Westwood (1984) points out, it has long been assumed that pregnancy, childbirth and motherhood are matters related to family life and to women at home, rather than the workplace. In the past this assumption has meant that these issues have not been well addressed within organisations. This may also partly explain why issues to do with sexuality have long been ignored at work. In recent years, many organisations have started to face the realities of dual career couples, women with children returning to work and individuals prioritising family and other commitments above work. This has triggered greater interest in achieving a work–life balance and increasing interest in people's relationships and other commitments (*Diversity Challenge* 2000). However, change is slow and generally speaking emotional, family and sexual issues are still sidelined within work.

Where work takes place

The opposition of emotions, sexuality and the personal with work is premised upon a particular view of work. Indeed, it could be argued that it is a very gendered view. Dorothy Smith suggests that were we to start from the position of women in the home, the apparent contrast between these two spheres would not make sense: 'The social organisation of the roles of housewife, mother and wife does not conform to the division between being at work and not being at work' (Smith 1988:68). Moreover, a number of writers have argued that women experience their lives in a more holistic way than the model of separate spheres suggests. Davidoff and Westover (1986) for example, suggest that women tend to mesh employment with domestic commitments. However, the situation may be more complex. For, as Finch points out in work on wives' incorporation into men's work, some women's lives in fact are organised to fit around their husbands' work (1983:1). Home-based work in particular changes the character of the relationship between work and non-work time, undermining the notion of separate spheres. As Finch states: 'Where work is based in the home the home is part of the 'public' domain, both structurally and experientially and the notion that there is a clear distinction between the two is called into question' (Finch 1983:58).

As well as those working at home, there are people whose living and workspace is the same, for example those in the army. Hearn and Parkin (1987) describe such places as total institutions and suggest that they are the environments where the more usual division between the private–public domain is redrawn, blurred or even abolished. Where there is a physical separation between home and work, the spheres may still be bridged, for example, by talking about work at home. It may

therefore be misleading to suggest any individual or occupational group is characterised either by similarity between home and work or by contrast; some features
of work will be replicated and others contrasted.

Sex as leisure

One of the important features of past sociological work has been the equation of
sex with personal life and leisure. For many, sex is clearly seen as part of personal
life. Wives, for example, may experience their husbands' work affecting their sex
life as an intrusion: 'It's pretty bad when you get in bed and you're making love
and you hear the g-d- phone ring. It interrupts arguments, it interrupts meals, but
sex is the ultimate of interruptions' (Fowlkes in Finch 1983).

The ideology of separate spheres, or perhaps separate activities at separate
times, is clearly at play again, when, ' "The long arm of the job" stretches from the
workplace into the bedroom and exerts its grip on the most intimate part of marriage' (Luxton 1980:55).

Terms such as 'the ultimate' and 'most intimate' here suggest that sex is strongly
associated with the personal. However, there is also a recognition that work crosses
personal boundaries in its effects on sex. For example, Duncombe and Marsden
(1995) have discussed the effects of work on couples, including their sex lives,
although only in terms of heterosexuality. This is also true of research by Devaney
(1991) on miners, which describes the impact of men's shiftwork on their sex lives.
Other references to the impact of work on 'home and family' often contain implicit
reference to sex and Lippert's (1977) work makes this explicit. In an article on
working in a car plant, he describes how he experiences a link between work and
sex, arguing that his work affects his sexuality at 'home'. Lippert (1977) asserts
that because his work was asexual or anti-sexual he needed more sex and his sexuality became more genitally focused. This is not an isolated account. Nickolay also
refers to work having affected his sexual behaviour: 'I would come home feeling
so dead that I masturbated to bring some life back to me. In the last four weeks I
would masturbate at work in the toilets – it refreshed me, I came a little bit alive in
myself' (Nickolay 1991:161).

The idea that boring work creates a need for sex is of course too simplistic, and
the idea that sexuality is ignored because it is unprofitable does not stand up to
empirical investigation. For example, Roy (1974) observed how managers used
harassment or flirtation strategies to get women to work harder, and work by
Halford *et al.* (1997) suggests that management supported flirtation and sexual
banter at work because it was felt to be productive, although within limits. However, what both Nickolay and Lippert suggest is that people often experience work,
leisure and home as interdependent. Indeed Luxton (1980) has argued that
increased cultural emphasis on the importance of sexuality can affect people's
experience of work and leisure by making sex more central to their leisure activities. Her account also suggests a need to consider how sex may affect work. She
writes that older men often tease younger men at work for being lazy, saying it is
because they are tired from having had so much sex.

The private in the public

One of the main problems with the idea of public–private spheres is that this opposition neglects the fact that there are private aspects of work. In an account of factory life, Westwood (1984) describes the elaborate rituals surrounding weddings and brides, which meant that company time and resources were used not for profit, but for women on the shop floor. Workers' rights to this time and these resources were acknowledged by management, who knew from experience that if they attempted to intervene in these spaces they would have 'a walk off' (1984:90). In the same way, management accepted aprons being made in company time, with company material, because they knew that women had to do work which left fluff on their clothes. Westwood suggests that through these practices the women were able to 'feminise' the masculine world of work:

> Aprons brought the world of the home and of domestic labour right into the middle of the factory and by so doing they extracted from the company something much more than their fabric pieces and the labour time involved in their production. They brought the world of home into the factory.
>
> (Westwood 1984:22)

Elsewhere, workers may sometimes be allowed to undertake certain domestic duties at work, for example making personal phone calls, although this is usually within limits. Friendship at work and discussion of personal issues offers another example of how private and public spheres are integrated (Seidler 1991; Westwood 1984). Certainly, places that are less directly controlled by management provide opportunities for meeting, intimacy and even sexual behaviour (Hearn and Parkin 1987).

There are also times when the private can become public, for example when leisure and homely pursuits have a work function, by networking, entertaining or getting to know colleagues. For example, Sheppard (1989) notes that women in management positions mention such places as bars, strip clubs, fishing trips and the golf course as areas from which they are in varying degrees excluded, but where they know that important organisational information is exchanged and decisions made.

These examples show that the situation is far more complex than any simple public–private distinction. Indeed, the ambiguity of terms such as 'private' and 'home and family' have often served to obscure rather than to reveal.

Sex and sexuality at work

Although early sociological work on organisations and professions neglected to discuss sex or sexuality, descriptions of working environments often revealed instances of harassment or sexual expression, even in occasional notes or comments. Hearn and Parkin (1987) give numerous examples. A study by Harrison (1943), for example, contains the following sexualised description: 'a lively very good looking girl of twenty with lovely naturally wavy hair, which she wears loose on her shoulders ... she always wears nice dresses and stockings to work, regardless of ... dirt and oil' (Harrison 1943:33–4).

Under the impact of the second wave of feminism, there has been greater recognition of women's experiences within organisations and, as a result, more specific writing about sex and sexuality at work. Much of this, however, has been in the form of sexual harassment studies. Research by the National Opinion Poll shows that most women at work will experience some form of sexual harassment (Kellner 1991) and this is supported in descriptions of working life (Cavendish 1982; Hearn and Parkin 1987; Pringle 1989; Secrett 1991).

A focus on the experiences of women has also highlighted the androcentrism of previous sociological studies. Feminists have shown that men's experiences are often written about as if they are universal, thus invisibilising gender differences. This gender blindness may be one reason why the sex–work opposition has held sway for so long, for it seems that women are less likely to experience a separation of sex and work than men. As Pringle asserts:

> For women the two obviously go together ... . Women are constantly aware of sexual power structures and the need to put up barriers against men (at work). Though they enjoy male company and male jokes they are careful to limit their participation and to make it clear to men 'how far they can go'.
>
> (Pringle 1989:163–4)

In her work with secretaries she reports:

> Male bosses can decide for themselves the extent to which they will keep home and work, their public and private lives separate. Secretaries do not have this luxury. Male bosses go into their secretaries' offices unannounced, assume the right to pronounce on their clothes and appearance, have them doing housework and personal chores, expect them to do overtime at short notice and ring them at home ... men 'invade' women's private space all the time and women have to defend it. The sexual metaphor is apt.
>
> (Pringle 1989:169)

The specificity of women's experiences has also been highlighted by Sheppard who shows how female managers often have to 'blend in' to conform to the prevailing expectations and comfort levels of male co-workers and bosses. She argues that women have constantly to maintain a delicate balance between being feminine enough, yet business like. Women are caught in a double bind, for:

> femaleness embodies sexuality which must be contained, but being seen as 'unfemale', i.e. not sexually attractive or available to men (for example a lesbian) still means that a woman is perceived primarily in sexual terms.
>
> (Sheppard 1989:147)

Other writers have noted the pressure on women to hide their bodies. For example Laws (1990) has discussed the need for women to adopt a 'menstrual etiquette' (whereby menstruation is hidden from others) at work, and Sheppard offers some extraordinary examples of advice from books designed to help working women. These include statements such as 'There's only one lingerie rule for the business-woman: Wear bras that hold your breasts in place and hide your nipples' (Molloy in Sheppard 1989:150). Such examples suggest that men and women may experience their sexuality in very different ways at work, and are expected to manage their bodies in distinct ways.

The sociological recognition that sexuality as an organisational phenomenon is wider than the issue of harassment came with key publications such as *Sex at Work* (Hearn and Parkin 1987) and *The Sexuality of Organisation* (Hearn *et al.* 1989). These books built on feminist studies of sexual harassment, together with organisational theory, to explore neglected issues of sex and sexuality. They emphasised that sexuality plays an important, if often unrecognised, role in work relationships and that organisations are not places exempt from sex and sexuality.

Although most people do not have sex where they are employed, sexual behaviour does occur in organisations, and takes many forms such as: sexual display, exploitation of sexuality, sexual advances and horseplay (Hearn and Parkin 1987). Several writers have highlighted the pervasive nature of sexuality at work:

> Sex is like paperclips in the office: commonplace, useful, underestimated, ubiquitous. Hardly appreciated until it goes wrong. It is the cement in every working relationship. It has little to do with sweating bosses cuddling their secretaries behind closed doors ... It is more adult, more complicated, more of a weapon.
>
> (Jones 1972:12)

How is sex at work expressed?

Early accounts of sex and sexuality at work often took their examples from life in factories. For example, Roy (1974) mentions: derogatory comments from male workers about having had sex with their female co-workers; how the ending of love affairs affected production; sexual harassment; and male supervisors deliberately using flirtation or harassment to get women to work. He argues that sex is not a taboo topic in the blue-collar world, so long as interaction is kept strictly verbal. Restraint is only exercised over its duration. Lippert (1977) describes how he was struck by the kind of role sexuality plays in mediating relationships. He documents an intense pressure to compete with other men in terms of exhibiting sexual experience and competency. He also describes physical contact between men, although he notes that this is not usually considered sexual.

Although there has been some recognition of the importance of male homosociality at work (Kanter 1977; Thompson and Ackroyd 1994), it is interesting how many people assume sex only occurs when men and women are together. Several writers have discussed the 'problematic' nature of male and female work groups, arguing that they engender a sexualised atmosphere. Bryant (1974) suggests that mixed sex groups create an over concern for appearance, jealousy and flirtation that leads to bad work performance. He claims it is for this reason that rules and social norms about sex are constructed. His at times obsessive focus on mixed work groups and the sex it is assumed this causes seems misguided because his analysis appears to sexualise *all* encounters between men and women. By way of contrast, work by Halford *et al.* (1997) suggests that staff and managers often prefer mixed sex groups because they improve performance. They are described as less 'laddy' or 'bitchy' and seen to contain and constrain excessive sexual discussion.

Accounts of working life often reveal examples of sex and sexuality, even when this is not their prime focus. References include gossip and discussions about sex and romance; sexual harassment; flirtation; jokes about sex; sexual rituals; sexual relationships; sexual pictures; and physical contact (Cavendish 1982; Devaney 1991; Halford *et al.* 1997; Secrett 1991; Westwood 1984). Although Hearn and Parkin (1987) also acknowledge many of these examples, they write that sexuality is always: 'one step removed from being pinned down' because it is usually expressed in subtleties, gossip, joking, rumours or innuendo. Although this may be true in some cases, sex is not always hidden or secret. Indeed Halford *et al.* (1997) state that many of their interviewees readily discussed issues related to sexuality when talking about the impact of changing gender roles. The tendency within the existing literature to see sex and sexuality at work only in terms of gossip, harassment or sexual banter does little to help illuminate the experiences of those such as the outreach workers described in this study, who are working in a field where sex and sexuality is an openly acknowledged part of work.

Most published examples of sex and sexuality at work focus on heterosexuality; much less research appears to have been conducted with lesbians and gay men. Where non-heterosexual experience is discussed it is usually in relation to coming out in the workplace (Rust 1993), or the difficulties faced in working in heterosexual environments (Hall 1989). Few writers point out that the masculinities they are discussing are usually heterosexual ones, or consider what this might mean for their analysis. In fact, where authors have described homosocial work contexts, they rarely question the sexuality of the men or women within them, and therefore neglect to address the diverse ways in which sexuality may be expressed at work.

Sexual skills

There has been a growing recognition that some relationships and occupations are themselves sexualised through organisational structures and relationships. This has led some writers to argue that personal qualities, interpersonal skills, and the physical appearance of workers are used through the employment of specific sexual or emotional skills within the workplace. For example, Hochschild (1983), in a now famous book *The Managed Heart*, discusses the experience of female flight attendants who were taught various forms of impression management to ensure they are always smiling and attractive towards their customers. Knights and Morgan (1991) and Halford *et al.* (1997) have also noted the value of employing 'attractive' women in clerical work or at the front of organisations. Research by Adkins (1992) on women in the tourist industry has further developed these ideas. She describes how:

> Within tourist employment women workers are recruited not simply on the basis of the particular skills or resources needed for particular jobs, but also on the basis of fulfilling a set of conditions relating to appearance ... . Not only were women required to have an attractive, pleasing appearance to be employed, but part of the women's jobs ... involved the maintenance of their looks. Thus if the women looked tired, wore too little or too much make-up, or failed to wear their uniforms in the prescribed manner ... they were instantly warned to correct their appearance problems ... . For men in these organisations no such conditions were in operation.
>
> (Adkins and Lury 1994:16–17)

Adkins' (1992) recognition of the relationship of the sexual to the economic is very important. People are paid for their work-related skills, and some of these may be sexual. In this way sexuality and personal issues may be tied into economics.

Although there has been some recognition of how women come to undertake sexual and emotional labour, little work seems to have addressed how men's bodies may be used in this way. Part of the reason for this neglect is that men have traditionally been seen as 'unemotional' and therefore not involved in emotion work. However, as Craib states:

> It is important to realise that whatever stereotype an individual might appear to meet – whether the unemotional, frigid male or the warm, caring female – he or she will be engaged in intense emotional work. We are not talking about society allocating emotional labour to women; rather, men and women might engage in different forms of labour or might be assigned different ways of displaying their emotional behaviour. In this context apparently 'unemotional' behaviour is very emotional. The only truly unemotional behaviour I know of is death.
>
> (Craib 1995:155–6)

This is a very important point. As we will see later, outreach workers describe using their body (and cruising skills) within work and as such can be seen to engage in both emotional and sexual labour to mediate their relationships with service users.

Men often feel it necessary to engage in sexual banter to compete with each other and gain acceptance (Collinson and Collinson 1993), and gay male workers have discussed the strategies they use at work to pass as heterosexual (Bryson 1994). While men may not be expected to employ the same sexual skills as women, this does not mean they employ no sexual skills. Indeed, the fact that historically some organisations have preferred men to be married before they are promoted,[2] suggests that men's sexuality may perhaps be bought too, albeit in a very different way (Halford *et al.* 1997). Gutek suggests men may 'use their sexuality' at work more than women. The examples she gives include using sexuality to intimidate women, to elicit sexual overtures, to make sexual jokes or compliments, and to encourage women to work harder (1993:63–4). She argues that men may be more successful at using sexuality within work as such behaviour may be interpreted as ability for leadership, or to 'get the job done'. There is a need for more detailed analysis of the use of sexuality and sexual skills by both men and women.

Pleasure or danger, sexuality or gender?

Much has been written about flirtation and joking relationships at work. Pringle (1989), for example, suggests that for men and women sexual fantasies and inter-actions are a way of killing time, of giving a sense of adventure, and livening up an otherwise boring day. Certainly, talk about sex seems to form a part of camarade-rie, which can be important. Cavendish (1982) writes that she and the factory workers chatted about everything under the sun including marriage and abortion, and Westwood (1984) reports that sex played a crucial ingredient in the many pic-tures and jokes which made factory work tolerable.

Talk about sex plays a role in maintaining friendships at work as well as provid-ing opportunities for enjoyment. It is for this reason that Pringle (1989) has argued that an overemphasis on sexual harassment has neglected the pleasure women may also gain from sexual interactions. Halford *et al.* (1997) also found that in some circumstances women enjoyed sexualised talk and flirtation, when it is clearly dis-tinct from harassment. This talk was felt to be exciting, partly because it was seen as something different to work. Despite the fun sexualised jokes and discussion may generate, it is important to note how limited an expression of sex and sexuality they seem to allow. Pringle points out how relentlessly heterosexual daily life in the office can be. She describes how a lesbian secretary she interviewed told her that: 'she deliberately chose temporary work so that she could move on before having to face the chit chat over morning tea about private life' (1989:165). It can also be unclear where the boundaries are between flirtation and sexual banter, and sexual harassment.

One of the problems caused by the heterosexual focus of much existing research is that writers sometimes use the term sexuality when it appears they are discussing gender relations. The conflation of sexuality and gender means that issues of sexu-ality have often been reduced to gender, which neglects and ignores the unique experiences of lesbian, gay and bisexual workers, as well as their relationships with heterosexuals. Furthermore, the term sexuality is sometimes used to cover sexual attraction, relationship status, parental status and almost any contact involv-ing the body. There is clearly a need for less vagueness and for more sophisticated definitions.

Boundaries

When sex and sexuality have been addressed in the literature, few authors have looked at how people draw boundaries at work in relation to sexual matters. Elsewhere in the literature sexual boundaries have been discussed in relation to sex between therapists and clients, and other professionals involved in similar trusting relationships. Rutter (1991) in a book on exploitative sexual relationships writes:

> It took me nearly a decade to stop believing in the myth of the beneficent doctor. I discovered instead that sexual exploitation by men of women under their care or tutelage is not unusual and in actuality is quite common. Furthermore, I found remarkably similar patterns of sexual contact not only by male doctors and therapists but by male clergy, lawyers, teachers and workplace mentors. These highly eroticised entanglements can occur, behind closed doors, in any relationship in which a woman entrusts important aspects of her physical, spiritual, psychological, or material welfare to a man who has power over her ... . I can see now that sexual violation of trust is an epidemic, mainstream problem that re-enacts in the professional relationship a wider cultural power-imbalance between men and women.
>
> (Rutter 1991:1–2)

He argues from a psychological and cultural perspective that therapeutic relationships, although meant to be protective, often become intensely erotic leading to many men ignoring the moral, legal and ethical responsibilities of their professions and engaging in sexual relationships with their female clients. Having professional codes does not necessarily deter sex taking place, and indeed for some members may even psychologically encourage it by presenting this sex as forbidden.

In recent years, there has been a steady stream of books addressing the issues of professionalism and sexual boundaries, though mostly written in an American context, e.g. Friedman and Boumil 1995; Gonsiorek 1995; and Snipe 1995. There have also been international conferences on Sexual Misconduct by Clergy, Psychotherapists, and Health Care Professionals, and the breaking of sexual boundaries has come to media attention as a widescale problem. In the UK there has been discussion about the need to develop codes of conduct for university lecturers (*Times Educational Supplement* 1995), and a conference in 1993 addressed this issue (Brookman 1993). In the USA, sexual liaisons with priests and parishioners are reported to have become a major public scandal (Francoeur 1996). Some dioceses even fear bankruptcy because of the amount of damages they have had to pay out to survivors of abuse by Catholic priests (Francoeur 1996). Perhaps the most recent public discussion of sexual boundaries in the USA arose with revelations about the sexual relationship between President Clinton and Monica Lewinsky.

Increasing reports of 'sexual misconduct', and discussions about the need for codes of conduct and boundary making, can be seen as part of a wider interest in sexual issues. Plummer (1995) argues that the increase in the number of sexual stories now being told highlights how traditional notions of public and private are breaking down. Increasingly prevalent accounts of private pain, for example, in stories of rape, sexual abuse or 'coming out' as lesbian or gay mean that:

> the most personal and private narratives have become the most public property. The domains of public and private have crumbled … the mass media has become a key story teller of our personal sexual lives in ways that even thirty years ago would have been inconceivable.
>
> (Plummer 1995:8–9)

Sexual boundaries have particular relevance for gay and bisexual men. For example, 'coming out' at work is a clear way in which public and private boundaries may be breached (Plummer 1995; Schneider 1986). Furthermore, in some occupations lesbians and gay men may find their private sex life is seen as making them unfit for work (Grey 1993; Rubin 1992). Perhaps in consequence, gay men not infrequently find their sexuality 'at the crossroads of the public and private' (Edwards 1994:3).

Boundary development and maintenance extends well beyond the domain of trusting relationships. Roy describes how people tend to compartmentalise many of their everyday activities: 'since work, recreation, art, religion and family life must be kept separate in time and place' (1974:45). However, he says little about how this is achieved. Halford *et al.* (1997) have discussed home and work boundaries and make some headway in analysing how people manage these. However, most of their discussion is focused around marriage, children and family commitments and so sheds little direct light on the experiences of those with other living arrangements such as the gay and bisexual outreach workers in this study. Importantly, however, they do mention the use of boundaries within work, for example in terms of self-presentation and the limits placed on discussion of emotional and personal issues at work. As they state, everyone made decisions about who it was appropriate to share personal issues with and worked hard to maintain a professional image: (1997:29, see also McElhinny 1994).

The need to draw boundaries between work and personal life[3] is raised by Cruikshank (1989) in an article on burnout amongst community development workers. She describes the difficulties involved in living, and working, in the same community and outlines how, through experience, workers learned the importance of meeting their own needs, and found ways to withdraw from work to spend time alone or with families. Although she does not use the term 'boundaries', she does describe some of the methods workers used to prevent burnout. These included individual coping methods like taking vacations or making lifestyle changes, social support systems including listening and supervision, and institutional practices such as teamwork and sabbaticals.

Professions and professionalism

The professions have long been of interest to sociologists. As Freidson notes:

> the professions have been singled out as occupations that perform tasks of great social value because professionals possess both knowledge and skills that in some way set them apart from other kinds of workers.
>
> (Freidson 1984:2)

Before the 1960s, most work on professions was bound up with discovering those characteristics which distinguished them from other occupations (Goode 1957; Greenwood 1957). However, all this work did not lead to a consensus. Freidson wrote that in 1972 it was hard to find agreement on the definition of a professional, despite the fact that this had been the subject of heated debate since at least 1915 (Freidson 1983). He argued for a focus instead on defining what was meant by the term 'professional' rather than trying to produce a single definition. A similar view has been pursued by Dingwall (1979) who suggests analysing the way members of different occupations use the term in their everyday activities. In this book, I explore professionalism in this way by looking at what the concept meant to HIV prevention outreach workers, and how being professional created tensions at the level of their everyday experience.

Over the past fifteen years, there has been a growing interest in the issue of professionalisation, or the process by which occupations turn themselves into professions, and what enables or impedes their claims to this status. This interest in how occupations control, and manage, a claim to special knowledge and privilege has led to work which addresses the ways in which professions protect their work from the encroachment of other occupations, and maintain their favoured position in the market. According to Larson (1977) the 'professional project' describes the processes by which members of a profession seek monopoly in the market and status in the social order. Members have to work to gain their status and then find ways to maintain and enhance their position. As part of this process, individuals must be socialised into the norms and values of the profession and be concerned with maintaining an image of respectability and trustworthiness. This is particularly important in securing their status both among clients and the wider public. To ensure that they alone have access to certain specialised knowledge and markets, professions use strategies of social closure (Witz 1992). This may involve entrance exams, qualifications and battles with other occupations over the boundaries of expertise.

Work on the professional project has highlighted the importance of socialisation in the production of professionals. An emphasis on identity, behaviours and values is important in focusing attention on the practices of professionals but is rarely discussed in detail. One notable exception is the work of Dingwall (1979) on how health visitors 'accomplish profession'. He describes how health visitors are trained in a range of behaviours, which enables them to enact a style of working which conveys the importance of their service. May *et al.* (1996) also address the more micro aspects of professional practice, in an article which explores the relationship between general medical practitioners and their patients. They argue that the everyday medical work of doctors reflects their professional rhetoric about the limits of and possibilities in relationships with patients. This argument is explored in two case studies, which highlight how different ideas about the nature of this relationship, for example as a therapeutic interaction, or in meeting the needs of a consumer, affect the way that the interaction is negotiated. Although they make mention of issues such as the length of consultations, the content of discussions, management of emotions and the focus of doctors on the medical aspects of patients' problems, these techniques are not really examined in detail.

Fahey's (1995) work in family studies offers some interesting examples of how ideas and rules relating to professional conduct can be seen to be related to public and private boundaries. He notes that some professional services cut across what is thought of as the public–private divide. Thus the priest, doctor, bank manager or solicitor all have access to highly personal information which may even be kept private from other family members. This means that the professional emphasis on trust, respectability and confidentiality take on special importance. This same phenomena has been noted by Robinson in his work on doctors:

> At whatever level, physical, biomedical, psychological or emotional, the doctor, in order to perform his professional role, is inevitably going to be involved in significant 'private' affairs of his patients.
>
> (Robinson 1973:74)

Furthermore, Robinson argues that because, as part of their role, doctors touch and investigate bodies, there is a need for them to justify their behaviour through adherence to a professional role. As we shall see later, the sexualised nature of outreach work and the need to justify one's role to others were some of the reasons why the workers in this study placed such emphasis on the need to be professional.

Sex and professionalism

Issues related to sex and sexuality are almost entirely absent in research on the professions. It is significant that in the whole of Macdonald's (1995) *The Sociology of the Professions*, which provides an excellent summary of the main literature in this area, there is not a single mention of sexuality. Elsewhere in the literature, occasional oblique references can be found, such as Paterson's (1983) point that at one time divorcees were excluded from the bench, and references to the need for professionals to maintain decorum in their private lives, but rarely is there any substantive discussion of sexuality. The fact that the sociological literature is so silent on this issue is interesting given that references to sexual conduct can often be found in professional guidelines and codes of conduct. However, the fact that professional guidelines often attempt to regulate the sexual behaviour of their members also demonstrates how sex and sexuality are seen as antithetical to professionalism. This raises interesting issues about how those involved in sex-related work can maintain their professional status. Certainly, within the existing literature one can find numerous examples of professionals facing difficulties because of the sexuality and sex-related nature of their work (Udry 1993; Ussher 1993; Vance 1991). However, these issues rarely cross over into the literature on professions. Neither is there much work addressing the relationship of sexuality to the professional project, despite important work regarding gender. One of the interesting aspects of this particular study, then, lies in its exploration of how those in an occupation which by its very nature could be seen to be unprofessional, relate to ideas of professionalism.

Sexuality and organisations

As Gutek (1989) and Rutter (1991) have noted, it is important to see sexuality and sexual behaviour as integral to organisational structures and the work environment. Such an emphasis helps to shift the focus towards the relationship of sex and sexuality to power in organisations, and recognises the links with wider social relationships. As Hearn and Parkin (1987) argue, sexuality needs to be seen as an ordinary and frequent public process, rather than a separate and discrete set of practices. The ways in which sex and sexuality are expressed at work, and the boundaries drawn between home and work, are not just a matter of individual preference. Organisations favour certain patterns of accommodation between home and work life. This is usually one that relies on a stereotypical gendered division of labour, and to which it has been easier for men to conform.

The idea that sex at work has to be controlled in order for production to occur forms part of what Foucault terms 'the repressive hypothesis': namely, the idea that sex must be rigorously repressed because it is incompatible with a general and intensive work imperative (1981:6). For Foucault (1981) however, power is about more than censorship, prohibition and denial. It triggers a multiplicity of resistances and cultural forms. Importantly, as we shall see, outreach workers actively constructed guidelines about sex with their managers and some used their sexuality in work as a way to challenge organisations.

Part of the power of sexuality in organisational contexts arises from an ambiguous interplay with the supposedly desexualised world of organisations and work (Hearn and Parkin 1987). Indeed Foucault notes that if one sees sex as repressed, then the mere fact of speaking about it takes the form of deliberate transgression:

> For decades now we have found it difficult to speak on the subject without striking a different pose: we are conscious of defying established power, our tone of voice shows that we know we are being subversive.
>
> (Foucault 1981:7)

No doubt this is why some have seen displays of sex and sexuality at work as a strategy of resistance (Burrell 1984). In another factory study, Pollert (1984), for example, described how women used their femininity and sexuality as a means of confronting management controls and the sexism of male supervisors. However, this meant colluding in the definition of woman as sex object. For this reason, she felt that shop floor culture was a form of symbolic resistance, which remained at the level of style, rather than developing into organised resistance to exploitation.

Burrell (1984) has argued that the control of sexuality is a major formal preoccupation of bureaucracy, and certainly organisations do much to control the physical and emotional distance and proximity between people. This in turn affects the sexual expression between organisational members and, I would suggest, between them and clients. Organisations may also institutionalise sexuality through professional codes and regulations. However, such regulations may be as much about acquiring professional status or maintaining an image of professionalism as a simple desire to improve work performance and save time.

It is clear that methods of exerting control over sex and sexuality vary across organisations and workplaces. The more broad minded and sympathetic organisations are to the person's total life situation, including their domestic arrangements, the more the private and sexual aspects of people's lives become a legitimate concern of organisations. Hearn and Parkin (1987) argue that with the emergence of human relations theory, management could legitimately take a more complete view of the worker including their emotional life and 'personal situation'. While this created the possibility of a more sympathetic and responsive management, it also expanded opportunities to patronise and manipulate workers. Silverman (1991) and Knights and Morgan (1991) both suggest that organisations and management benefit from personal information about workers.

Like sex and sexuality, there has been a limited consideration of emotion in organisation theory. Fineman (1991) suggests that this has led to thinking and writing about work and organisations which often bears little semblance to people's everyday experience. He suggests that emotions are totally caught up in activities and roles within work, and argues that powerful people can determine what is emotionally 'correct' for the enterprise, forcing a harsh split between what people feel and what they feel they can show. Work is often structured and performed according to specific rules, for example legal codes and informal social norms, some of which are external to the occupational or work system. Indeed, Smith (1988) and Pringle (1989) argue that the apparent neutrality of rules and goals disguise the class and gender interests served by them. We need, therefore, to look at the extent to which sexuality is expressed or repressed within organisations and where it is expressed, ask whose interests are dominant. Certainly the picture is more complex than a simple repression or resistance of sexuality at work.

2 Reflexivity, identity and boundaries

Every journey conceals another journey within its lines: the path not taken and the forgotten angle.

(Winterson 1990:10)

Many of the dilemmas outreach workers described in relation to identity, boundaries and professionalism were mirrored in my own experience conducting the research (Deverell 1993). These included issues of confidentiality, the role of identity in building rapport and the impact of the work on social and sexual life. Even some of the techniques used to collect information were similar, such as gaining credibility, securing access, developing relationships and making decisions about when to self disclose. Here, I will explore some of these issues through a discussion of the design of the study and the factors that shaped its development. A reflexive approach is adopted both to show how the research was carried out and to reflect on issues that influenced the process of enquiry as it unfolded.

The toolbox

The backbone around which the analysis was developed consisted of twenty-five semi-structured, in-depth individual interviews. However, I also co-facilitated a day workshop on boundary maintenance in HIV work, undertook some participant observation as a sessional outreach worker and analysed written documents. In addition my experience working in, and advising on, HIV prevention work with gay and bisexual men informed the work immensely (see Figure 1).

Individual interviews

Twenty-five people in total were interviewed. The majority (21) were gay or bisexual men. All worked in HIV prevention, and had undertaken work with a community outreach component. At the time of interview two of the men were still directly involved in HIV prevention, but one had just become a manager of an outreach programme and the other was involved in more general health promotion activities.

Main methods employed

- 25 in-depth semi-structured interviews lasting an hour or more
- Workshop on boundaries in HIV work
- Participant observation: 7 months paid, part-time sessional outreach work. Steering group member, trainer and researcher on various gay men's HIV prevention projects
- Documentary analysis

Sampling for interviews

- Purposive sampling of 25 paid HIV prevention outreach workers
- Personal contact and snowballing
- Workers interviewed from 10 areas of England

Demographic and social characteristics of interviewees

- 18 gay men, 3 bisexual men, 3 lesbians, 1 heterosexual woman
- Age range 22–50, most mid-twenties to thirties
- Five men were from black or ethnic minority communities
- All undertook HIV prevention with gay men, using outreach techniques
- Interviewees included 4 managers of outreach work

- 8 workshop participants (1 woman and 7 gay men)

Figure 1 Methods and sample.

I also interviewed one person who had a long history of carrying out and managing outreach work but was no longer undertaking it. He had, however, recently run a training course on boundary development and maintenance.

Although the focus of the study was on gay and bisexual male outreach workers, I interviewed some women as a form of theoretical sampling. This enabled me to draw out issues in the men's experiences related to gender and sexuality. Many of the issues related to boundaries were common to both male and female workers, but issues specifically to do with sexual boundaries were most acute for (single) gay and bisexual men. All of the women interviewed undertook outreach work with gay, bisexual and homosexually active men. Two of these women also worked with other groups. Although the number of women interviewed was small, occasionally I have used examples from their experiences within the book to help highlight key themes and issues.

Interviewees varied in age from 22–50, but the majority of them were in their mid-twenties to thirties. Five men came from black or minority ethnic groups and I interviewed people working in ten different areas of England. Some workers were new to post, and others had been undertaking outreach work for a long time. Given that workers talked about learning over time to draw boundaries, this difference turned out to be useful. I have not included much demographic data about those I interviewed because the small and networked nature of the HIV prevention field makes confidentiality a vital issue. In this way, my concerns were similar to those of the workers struggling to maintain their own personal and professional boundaries (see Chapters 5 and 6). I have used fictitious names throughout and only identify the part of the UK the worker was based in.

Participant observation

I was directly involved in HIV prevention work from 1988 to 1998 and throughout the time I was involved in this study I had other jobs in the HIV prevention field, mostly related to work with gay and bisexual men. This meant that I was constantly accumulating knowledge, which informed the work. Indeed, it was often frustrating that boundary issues would come up in circumstances where I was not formally researching. For example, I often heard interesting comments when sitting on interview panels, in casual conversations and office talk, or while undertaking other research or training. I usually felt unable to record this information and would not actively take notes or use material gathered in social or informal situations. However, such information contributed to my understanding of the political context and pressures on outreach. It enriched both the collection and analysis of data.

Participant observation took several forms and varied from complete participation to complete observation, with most of my experience being somewhere in the middle. It included seven months as a part-time, paid, sessional outreach worker; three years as evaluation fieldworker for a national community-based HIV prevention project; being a Trustee of a gay and bisexual HIV prevention organisation in London; sitting on the steering group of a Men who have Sex with Men health promotion project in the Midlands; discussion with workers in the HIV prevention field at conferences, etc.; membership of evaluation advisory groups for several gay men's projects; evaluating a national HIV Prevention Roadshow project, and conducting regional workshops with gay men's workers.

The paid outreach work involved total participation. This work took place with students in two higher education establishments and involved setting up health information stalls and handing out condoms, lubricant, Femidoms and information at social events. Throughout this time, I kept a personal diary in which I recorded boundary-related issues that came up for me. In this diary, I also made a note of issues that occurred in the evaluation of the HIV Prevention Roadshow project. Part of this evaluation involved helping to staff Roadshow stalls in a young offenders' institute, a hospital and a gay pub. All of this experience was useful in enabling me to gain insight into the work of those that I interviewed. I saw the experience of participant observation not as placing myself in the position of others but more as enabling me to better appreciate their feelings and experiences. In this way I tried to use and reflect upon my own experiences and emotional reactions (Kleinman 1991; Wright-Mills 1983), and I include some of these in the book.

In Helen Chadwick's (1994) art exhibition 'Effluvia' were some of her 'Viral landscape' photographs. These combined scenic landscapes of cliffs and the sea overlaid with pictures of Chadwick's own body cells. These pictures offer a powerful example of how, when studying something, one begins to see examples of it everywhere. As this study progressed I would find myself reading novels and underlining quotes which I thought were pertinent to the research; I would clip articles from newspapers; find my ears pricking every time I heard the phrase 'professional' on TV; and would come home from dinner parties wishing I had had my notebook to keep records of the conversation. This informal and formal participant observation was valuable because it gave me an opportunity to hear boundary issues being talked about in different settings and to see the reactions of managers and others to the issues being discussed. This meant that within interviews I could encourage detailed reflections on issues I had heard, seen or read and use these insights to explore processes that are less visible (for example psychological judgements and feelings).

Documentation

Hammersley and Atkinson (1993) argue that documentary analysis can be important because of the role written materials play in many organisations, particularly in relation to professionalism and organisational control (Kinsman 1997). Smith (1988) also notes that we are 'ruled through documents' and Latour (1990) has pursued this idea more theoretically in an article, which explores the role of documents in the creation and dissemination of 'facts'. Plummer (1995) also points to the importance of documentary analysis, although for a different reason. In his book *Telling Sexual Stories,* he claims that because of the way in which the media has become sexualised, printed materials are very important. I found that existing documentation was useful in providing background, context and further material to flesh out my ideas. Documents were often referred to in interviews and it was important to look at these for the details people could not remember. Written materials also proved useful in highlighting perspectives on boundaries that were *not* mentioned in interviews.

Early on in the research I was encouraged to discover the professional or trade journals relevant to the field and to read them. I puzzled at the time what might count as a trade journal for outreach workers. On reflection it was obvious: *The Pink Paper.* This is a national weekly newspaper for lesbians and gay men and at the time often carried articles on HIV prevention. Articles in this paper were frequently mentioned by outreach workers across the country and, for a while, it seemed that this was where many of the debates within the field emerged. The fact that some leading (London-based) figures in HIV prevention then had close links with the press – Edward King (regular articles for *The Pink Paper* and *Positive Times*), Simon Watney (columns in *Gay Times*) and Peter Scott (column in the *Gay Gazette*) – meant that the gay press became a key forum for debate about gay men's HIV prevention. It is interesting to note that amongst those interviewed, more individuals appeared to read *The Pink Paper* than any health education journal. Indeed, the gay press was the only information source spontaneously referred to. In this way community papers continued to play their early role as a place in which gay men found information about HIV (see Chapter 3), although with time new sources began to emerge as significant.

Workshop

Towards the end of the fieldwork, I was asked to organise and co-facilitate a workshop on boundary work for the Pan-London Gay and Bisexual Men's Workers' Forum. This was attended by eight people, one woman and seven gay men, none of whom I had interviewed. This proved to be a useful source of data collection because the group discussion provided me an opportunity to watch how people dealt with boundary issues and situations. It also enabled me to ask pertinent questions, and to check ideas with a larger and more varied group of people.

The networked nature of the HIV field: access and anonymity

Gaining access to people to interview was not a major problem. Having worked in HIV prevention for some time, I was already aware of networks of outreach workers and I started the research by approaching people I knew. I then used a snowballing technique, asking these initial contacts to suggest other workers who might be willing to talk. Sometimes this happened spontaneously, with people suggesting contacts during the course of the interview. Several men also offered themselves as interviewees once they had heard about my research because they felt that the subject was so interesting. This gives a somewhat different slant to Van Maanen's observation that: 'Informants select the researcher as much as the researcher selects them' (1991:36). I only followed up one of these approaches, however, partly because I had secured enough contacts. Finding women to interview was slightly more difficult because there are few female outreach workers working in gay men's projects.

Obviously, this method of sampling brings its own sources of bias. I was particularly concerned because I knew many of those I initially interviewed, even if it was only a vague work-related acquaintanceship. I therefore decided that it was important to try and talk to people with whom I did not have an existing relationship. However, finding workers I did not know at all proved extremely difficult. I remember my initial dismay when I travelled to meet two men working on a project with which I had no previous contact only to find that they had been in a workshop I had given. The issue of being known also brought up boundary issues for me: could I include in the sample people I already knew? A colleague hearing this dilemma advised me to use the situation as data. He suggested that it showed how networked and 'cliquey' the field was, which in turn helped explain why boundary issues often emerge. By the end of the research, the sample was quite diverse in terms of the relationships I had had with people. It included individuals with whom I had no previous contact; people I had never formally met before but who knew of me; those I did not know at the time I interviewed but subsequently ended up working with; people I vaguely knew; and those I had worked with a lot before.

Many seemed enthusiastic about taking part and stated that the work was important, interesting and useful. Indeed, one manager from a project I approached said he was glad someone was addressing this issue, and many men said they would be delighted to take part. Not only was this helpful, it also highlighted how the issue was seen as important at the time. People were keen to express their views on a subject which was topical, and had at times been a source of major debate.

One of the things which helped in gaining access was having been involved in HIV prevention for some time. This provided some credibility, as I was not seen as an 'outside academic' but as a colleague or peer. Indeed, many of those I did not know were aware of the work I had been involved in, and this perhaps helped with access. In this way, I used my identity as an HIV worker or 'someone in the know' to gain access. Part of my credibility and acceptance as a researcher came from the personal and political motivation for doing the work that I shared with many of the workers. This emphasis on personal commitment was a predominant theme in the HIV field at the time, and those not 'truly committed to the cause' were often looked down upon or mistrusted. Trust seemed to be built on assumptions about personal values, commitment to HIV, and knowledge of gay slang and gay communities. This meant that it was my past experience, shared values and personal commitment that gave me credibility.

The importance of personal attributes and self-presentation applies in most qualitative research (Shaffir and Stebbins 1991). Certainly, the interactive nature of research means that people make assumptions about researchers' identities and motivations. This means that gaining access and credibility relies on negotiated definitions and understandings of the researcher's role:

> the researcher does not simply appropriate a particular status, but discovers that he or she is accorded a status by the hosts that reflects their understanding of his or her presence.
>
> (Shaffir 1991:79)

Any role has to be recognised and accepted as appropriate by participants if the researcher is to appear credible. Self-presentation is probably less of an issue when you are already known. As Narayan (1993) has pointed out, a pre-existing identity may subsume your presence as a researcher. The importance of previous experience, interest and motivation in doing a particular piece of research is not something that I have heard many other researchers highlighting as being important for gaining credibility. However, I imagine this to be the case. It may be that such issues are brought to the fore in HIV research because of the culture of personal commitment and distrust of professionals that has often seemed to exist (see Chapters 3 and 7).

As a past or present colleague, my relationship as a researcher was not always the main or only relationship I had with interviewees. Although I only interviewed people once, my relationship with them did not always begin or end with the interview itself. For example, I might have evaluated their work in the past, I might have sat on their interview panel or steering group, they might be on a steering group of mine, I may have been approached by them for advice on methodology or in doing outreach work, I might evaluate their work in the future, I may have had attended workshops and conferences with them, they might have read my work and I might have heard about theirs. Thus, at times, the research relationship took on the flavour of ethnography.

One of the advantages of having contact after the interview was that individuals kept me updated as to how their thoughts and feelings had changed. For example, one early interviewee told me he thought he had been too rigid about boundaries in the past and was now beginning to question some of his earlier ideas. This was useful in that it alerted me to the fact that boundaries are flexible and processual, and encouraged me to look at their development over time. With permission, I included in the analysis comments which respondents had made to me after the interview. I saw these interactions as adding perspective and, like Andrews (1991), thought it misguided to discount them simply because the tape recorder was not on.

Confidentiality, neutrality and self disclosure

One of the issues raised by knowing a lot of people in the field was confidentiality. Occasionally a worker would talk about a friend or colleague we both knew and, at times, it was obvious to me who was being discussed, something which interviewees were also aware of. In addition, people revealed personal information about themselves, for example, their experiences of sexual abuse, drug use or sexual relationships. Given that I was so involved in their area of work, it is surprising that people rarely expressed concerns about confidentiality. I was told work-related stories which people said they had not revealed to anyone else, and was given personal information about boyfriends and sex partners.

Similarly to Finch (1993), I found that most of those I spoke to appreciated having someone to talk to and found the interview enjoyable. Indeed many people said at the end: 'Enjoyed it, could talk for hours' or 'Thank you for that, I really enjoyed it.' In fact, it often seemed ironic that people who were clearly helping me would say things that suggested that I was doing them a favour. For example, the following is a quote from a letter I received giving feedback after an interview:

> It was very valuable and inspiring reading it (transcript) over now ... I can really see how far we've come ... . Thanks a lot for giving me the opportunity to participate, it's been very informative and useful. (Rachel, London)

It is interesting to consider what people gain from interviews. Things mentioned in the research included being able to talk about issues with someone not directly involved but who knew about the work; the opportunity to reflect on progress and what had been learned; the chance to discuss a personal concern or interest; the opportunity to use the interview to discuss other areas of concern (managers and organisational homophobia, funding, politics, management); seeing it as a form of supervision or confession; and seeking information from me.

Asking questions of me probably seemed quite natural to participants. Having been involved in similar work for some time, several people already knew, or knew of, me. This meant that occasionally people would seek my opinion on something or were curious about my views. People would also ask if I knew individuals they were discussing, or would ask me the name of someone they had forgotten. In this way they would highlight the shared knowledge we had.

Questions of neutrality and whether researchers should talk about themselves have been the subject of much debate, and there are different views on this matter (Baum 1988; Van Maanen 1991). Many, particularly feminist, researchers have suggested that personal involvement should not be equated with bias (Oakley 1981). Indeed researchers are encouraged to try and understand their impact rather than try and eliminate it. Silverman (1994) has argued from an interactionist perspective that interviews should be seen as social events rather than as about the production of authentic facts. In this way, the interview is about the interaction, or what Silverman describes as mutual participant observation. For this reason, he suggests it is important to look at the properties of interviews and analyse these rather than regard the interaction as a bias to be controlled or a distortion to be minimised.

Importantly, research 'neutrality' may itself be a form of relationship. Researchers' actions are subject to interpretation and so people will read motivations and meaning into detachment. For example, Singer (1993) suggests that this may be seen as a kind of side-taking. Indeed, when listening itself can have a major impact in making people feel valued it is difficult to see how one could be expected to produce a neutral reaction (Griffin 1991). I would usually only talk about myself if I felt it would move the conversation on or help people reflect on their own experiences. In addition, sometimes I was directly asked to talk and usually I did so: people clearly at times wanting or needing a reaction before they were willing to open up more.

Sometimes I used my own experience to ask questions, by relating what had happened to me or by using ideas developed through participant observation. Duck (1986) suggests that it is through intimate disclosure that trust is signalled, and this is obviously important in developing rapport. Interestingly, the concerns I had about how much information I should reveal about myself were often also mentioned by workers. Outreach workers often discussed the difficulty in expecting frankness and honesty if you were not being like this yourself but were keen to balance this with a focus on the needs of those they were working with.

Building research relationships is a process in which researchers are judged on their actions. Therefore, it is perhaps inevitable that issues relating to participation will occur. As Gans (1968) notes, people often forget why the researcher is there and expect them to participate and express feelings of interest. This means that researchers are put under pressure to involve themselves. Given this, researchers have to calculate the likely costs and benefits of making their own voices heard.

Being streetwise

Reading research methods textbooks I was surprised to discover the use of acceptable incompetence as a way of gathering data. This involves playing the role of the naive observer and sometimes asking 'dumb' questions (Fetterman 1991). This was a strategy I definitely did not use and it is interesting to consider why not. First, given that I had been involved in the HIV field for a long time, in fact longer than many of those interviewed, it might have looked odd if I had asked questions which made it appear I did not know about the context in which people were working. Indeed, remarks were often made to me in interviews such as: 'I'm sure you're aware'; 'as you'll know'; 'in this field we're both in', which indicated that people expected me to have some shared baseline knowledge. In addition, it was vitally important that as a heterosexual woman I made it clear that I did understand (rather than feign ignorance). This was particularly so because in interviews men often displayed anger about heterosexual managers not understanding their dilemmas; and consternation was sometimes expressed about heterosexuals in general. For this reason, it was important to be seen as one of the 'wise', something that other researchers have also found. As Agar notes:

> The second reason for not asking questions is that you should not have to ask. To be accepted in the streets is to be hip; to be hip is to be knowledgeable; to be knowledgeable is to be capable of understanding what is going on on the basis of minimal cues. So to ask a question is to show that you are not acceptable.
>
> (Agar 1980:456)

My need to be seen as credible also related to wider dynamics within the HIV field. There has often been criticism of people who are just in the field to make money, or for their career, rather than because of personal commitment. Playing the naive and clueless researcher could have reinforced unhelpful stereotypes of researchers as 'academics' not in touch with the real world, and lacking personal commitment to HIV prevention. My concern to appear informed did not mean, however, that I did not probe or seek clarification. Indeed, I tried to be rigorous in checking my own assumptions and interpretations. This was occasionally noticed by interviewees who would express mock shock at what I'd asked or joke about 'difficult questions'. For example the following extract shows the response to a question on how boundaries were made:

> *K:*   Right, how would you go about trying to do that?
>
> Well, how would I go about? Thanks for that question! Thank you so much. You're not meant to ask that! You're meant to just, you know, talk about, for about ten minutes about how one goes about setting these boundaries, not how *I* do it! (Keith, North)

Interestingly, many interviewees held a sophisticated understanding of the research process. People maintained some control over the information offered and the direction of interview, and some apologised for 'going off the subject'. They also displayed something of an awareness of research conventions, joking that they would have to speak in sentences so I could quote them *verbatim*, or telling me that I could include certain information if it was anonymised, otherwise I could use it to inform my analysis. In this way, interviewees themselves were aware of playing a role.

Walk it like you talk it: on not sharing identifications

A further methodological issue related to an important debate within the HIV field itself: namely, the re-gaying of AIDS (see Chapter 3). This process led to criticism from some people over the place of women in gay men's HIV prevention work, and exacerbated my anxieties about the appropriateness of my doing this work. The issue over who should research whom is a hotly debated methodological issue and parallels discussions among outreach workers themselves (see Chapter 7). These debates centre on whether only those with direct experience are able to contribute to an area (Hart 1993). Some feminists, for example, have suggested that in order to establish good rapport, only women should interview women (Finch 1993). The importance of shared identity is a difficult area, involving complex understandings of identity and identity politics.

Given my background, in some ways I felt I did share certain experiences with gay men doing outreach work. Indeed, interviewees often referred to me as someone who knew about the field and would share knowledge of topical issues and discuss well-known figures and debates. My knowledge of these areas, as well as an understanding of the gay scene and gay slang, was very useful in assisting interpretation and the development of rapport. In this way, my personal involvement in HIV prevention aided the research. However, it also raised questions about the kinds of experience needed to understand and develop rapport. My feeling was that developing a good research relationship did not necessarily demand sharing a specific gender or sexuality:

> Connections between interviewers and interviewees can be made through affirming whatever characteristics one or both parties may perceive themselves to hold in common.
>
> (Andrews 1991:56)

Indeed, it would have been impossible to interview twenty-five people and share identifications with all of them. For this reason, I find the idea that there should be a natural affinity between certain people too simplistic. For example, although Finch (1993) writes that women expected her to understand because she was another woman, I sometimes felt that gay men expected me to understand because of my experience researching HIV prevention. Indeed as Andrews again writes:

> While interviewer and interviewee may share certain group memberships (such as gender) they do not necessarily share others. It is important for the researcher to be sensitive to the way in which she is perceived by the partici- pant, as this will also influence the dynamics between the two people. Addi- tionally, the researcher interprets what is said to her through her own frameworks of understanding, which will invariably be influenced by her group memberships.
>
> (Andrews 1991:54)

It is for this reason that some writers have criticised the idea of 'natural' affinity (Cotterill 1992; Hammersley 1992). Indeed, this issue is one of wider theoretical concern (Brah 1992; Deverell and Prout 1995; Hall 1990; Haraway 1990).

How you are identified does, however, affect what you get told. Williams (1993) suggests that when researching the berdache tradition (in native American culture), being openly gay gave him access to informants and information about homosexuality among native Americans he would not otherwise have had. In an article on the influence of sex and gender on research Warren discusses her early fieldwork with gay men. She suggests that her gender restricted the kinds of places she could access, and information she could glean: 'An attractive male researcher could be able to document aspects of the world closed to a female' (Warren and Rasmussen 1977:65).

However, she also found that her gender and sexuality gave her access to privi- leged information, and points out how she:

> had access to areas of biographical experience less open to gay males because of the male sexuality focus of the world. Many of the gay men had had past sexual and marital experiences with women, which were rarely, or never a topic of conversation in the gay world. However, they were legitimate topics of conversation on a one-to-one interview basis with a female researcher with whom sexual interaction was not an issue.
>
> (Warren and Rasmussen 1977:356)

It therefore seems hard to predict what information will be revealed and what concealed. At times, being a woman may have prevented men from telling me cer- tain things. However, a number of the men interviewed suggested that because of a macho culture, it was quite difficult to talk about boundary issues or feelings with other gay men. This was particularly the case as they felt other gay men expected them to share certain points of view. Therefore, it may have been easier to talk about these feelings and difficulties to me.

Interestingly, I found that a shared gender did not automatically lead to easier rapport when interviewing women. Because I had interviewed and talked with more gay men on the subject of boundaries, and worked with gay men for a long time, I found that their experiences were more familiar to me. Although I managed to build rapport with the few women I interviewed, I certainly did not find it easier talking to them, as some other writers would suggest. This highlighted for me how complicated developing rapport is. It does not automatically occur just because people share a gender or sexuality. Indeed, individuals have more than one identity with which to relate to others, or with which to differentiate themselves. As Song and Parker highlight in an article relating to their experiences as mixed-race Chinese-English and Korean-American researchers interviewing Chinese young people in Britain:

> so many dimensions of sameness and difference can be operating at any given moment. And where two people may claim commonality on one dimension, they may fall apart on another.
>
> (Song and Parker 1995:246)

The fact that people have multiple identifications means that context is very important in determining how, when and why people will exercise a particular identity or identification (see Gatter 1993; Rhodes 1994a; Weeks 1990). Indeed the experiences of outreach workers reinforced the need not to take a simplistic approach to identity. Male workers spoke of the limitations of working around a shared gender and sexuality, and learned the need to address the diversity of men's feelings and experiences in their HIV prevention work, while all the female workers reported successfully working with a range of homosexually active men.

Protection and responsibility: presenting controversial work

Although for many researchers the act of writing marks the time when they leave, or have left the place of study, in many ways I have stayed attached. This means that I have been concerned both about what HIV prevention colleagues think about what I have written and also how the work will be used. My interest in the work being of practical use can be seen in the co-facilitation of the boundaries workshop, circulating papers I had written to interested workers and talking to interested individuals. Occasionally, interviewees used elements of this work themselves, for example in training or discussions with managers. My concern to make useful information available was tempered by a desire not to damage the reputation of outreach workers or subject them to even greater control.

One of the key challenges for me, as a straight woman writing predominantly about gay men, was not to exoticise those I had interviewed and worked with. Workers were very honest about their feelings and dilemmas and I was anxious to ensure that the subject of the study was not seen as titillating or trivial, but a serious issue. In part this concern was related to my recognition of the unusualness of this type of work and the desire to present outreach workers in a good light. This was an issue that workers themselves often also struggled with (see Chapter 3). My feeling of responsibility to those I had talked to meant that I was concerned to find ways of writing up the material that protected them and did not again lead to sensationalised media reporting of outreach work with gay men.

Another concern was to maintain the anonymity of those interviewed. For example, early on in the work I circulated a draft paper to ten interviewees and found that co-workers had been making guesses as to who the different quotes had come from. The fact that the HIV prevention field is so well networked, and that it would be relatively easy for others in the field to work out who was likely to have said what, meant that the fear of identifying someone was very real. For this reason, when quotations follow I have anonymised the speakers and also taken steps to prevent their identification from the area of the country they worked in.

A further issue for me involved deciding how much I should report my own boundary-related experiences. This is something raised by Clifford and Marcus (1986) who suggest that the questioning of objectivity by some social scientists has opened up a space for the publishing of more personal writing and a greater emphasis on the feelings and struggles involved in research. In terms of this book, it is interesting that this move has led to some anthropologists writing about the sexual experiences they have had when conducting ethnography (e.g. Abramson 1992; Kulick and Wilson 1995). Fowler and Hardesty (1994) suggest that because bringing personal issues into work has previously been regarded as unprofessional, anthropological and sociological researchers have only recently started to write about their personal experiences in fieldwork. This is particularly the case for those undertaking sex-related research, whose professionalism may already be tainted (Ussher 1996), and for whom writing about personal experiences can prove to be both damaging and risky. As Hart (1993) has noted, discussing her experiences from prostitution-related research, the subject of what you are studying plays a large part in how reflexive you can be. For this reason, the issue of personal and professional boundaries loomed large in the writing itself. In the book I have included a few examples of my own experiences where I think it aids discussion but I have chosen to keep the focus firmly on outreach workers' own experiences.

3 HIV prevention, gay communities and outreach work

There are many accounts of the history of the HIV epidemic. All are in some senses partial and incomplete, given its complexity and the fact that it has been experienced differently across the globe and within different communities (Bloor 1995; Davies *et al.* 1993; Holland *et al.* 1990). Many early accounts were based on US experience (Altman 1988; Shilts 1987; Patton 1985). This is not surprising given that the disease was first documented in the USA (CDC 1981).

What came to be termed HIV and AIDS was first recognised in 1981 when reports reached the US Centers for Disease Control (CDC) highlighting cases of gay men with a rare type of pneumonia (pneumocystis carinii, PCP) and a rare type of cancer (Kaposi's sarcoma, KS). This was seen as mysterious not only because both illnesses were unusual, but also because they were associated with severe immune deficiency; why were such diseases affecting young, healthy men? Soon reports of gay men with other opportunistic infections appeared and it became clear that underlying these infections was a severely impaired immune system. By 1982, this collection of clinical conditions, together with a suppressed immune system, had been given the status of a recognised syndrome: the Acquired Immune Deficiency Syndrome (AIDS).

Initially, medical scientists and doctors were unsure of the aetiology of the disease. Although early suggestions were that the disease was probably sexually transmitted, speculative theories concerning its causation abounded (Altman 1988; Patton 1985). Once the idea of a viral agent gained credence, there was a now famous chase between the French (Luc Montagnier) and Americans (Robert Gallo) to identify the virus responsible. The fact that this race ended in a court case highlights something of the economic and status factors resting on this scientific discovery. Subsequently, there was frenetic activity to discover a cause, cure and vaccine, with the lure of lucrative rewards. The virus responsible for AIDS was first isolated at the Pasteur Institute in Paris and confirmed to be a retrovirus. After several name changes HIV was announced in 1984 as being the cause of AIDS. Later different types of HIV were discovered which seem to have different virulences and are associated with different epidemics in different countries.

Many scientists and health promotion workers now talk about HIV disease (rather than HIV and AIDS), thereby explicitly recognising the underlying viral cause. While Peter Duesberg and others have put forward the idea that HIV is not the cause of AIDS (see Garfield 1994), a view given some credence by articles in some newspapers and by some AIDS activists (Positively Healthy, Gays Against Genocide), few others take it seriously. Most leading scientists agree that it is the action of HIV in destroying the immune system that results in the opportunistic infections that make up the syndrome AIDS. It is the presence of these infections that usually, and eventually, results in death.

Gradually, the increased availability of more sophisticated information about HIV and AIDS has helped the development of both prevention and treatment. In terms of prevention, the discovery that the main routes of transmission were through blood, semen and vaginal and cervical secretions led to the targeting of sexual behaviour and injecting drug use for prevention purposes. (There were also issues related to breast-feeding, blood transfusions and operations.) In relation to gay, bisexual and other men who have sex with men, the main source of transmission has been seen to be unprotected anal intercourse, although there is also an association with oral sex (Forbes 2000; Gorna 1996; King 1993a; King 2000). While there is still no cure and, as yet, no permanently effective way of controlling viral replication in an infected person, prevention is still seen as vitally important.

The British experience

The first British deaths of what was to become known as HIV and AIDS occurred in 1982. The realisation that men were dying mysteriously and suddenly in the USA, and that this might become a problem in Britain, was noted early on both by members of the gay community (usually those with friends, lovers or links to the USA) and medical scientists. In terms of the general public, it was documentaries such as the 'Killer in the Village' (BBC, Horizon 1983) that probably had most impact. The shock of this programme has been recalled by many (Davies *et al.* 1993; Edwards 1994) and I clearly remember seeing it while still at school.

It is hard to imagine now how intensely the tabloid press reacted to the emerging epidemic. Terrible homophobia, sensationalism and misreporting dominated the accounts focusing on the spread of the 'gay plague' to 'innocent victims'. A reaction against this was something that led to my own involvement in the field. It is also important to highlight the sense of panic and urgency many felt at that time. AIDS was initially portrayed as a terrible epidemic that would kill thousands. People had no idea what would happen and how many people were already infected. The sense of panic can be seen in the fears around kissing and sharing plates, and the 'space suits' and rubber gloves initially used when treating people with AIDS (Garfield 1994; Weeks 1991). In 1988, I was working in the post room at the Terrence Higgins Trust and remember seeing a leaflet especially designed to allay emerging fears about drinking from communion cups. This highlights the kind of panic caused by the paucity of information, and also shows how much more is now known.

The period between 1980 and 1986 has been characterised as a time of crisis, fuelled by media hype (Bennett and Ferlie 1994; Berridge 1992). Given the current normalisation of the epidemic now, and the associated low media profile (Needham 2000) it is easy to forget the sense of anxiety and uncertainty that then existed.

HIV prevention for gay men

'Well … my lover and I didn't split up. He died of AIDS.'
The kid blinked at him.
'Do you know what that is?'
Wilfred shook his head.
'It's this thing that gay men are getting in the States. It's a severe immune deficiency. They get it, and then they catch anything that flies in the window. Over a thousand people have died of it.' It felt strangely cold-blooded to start from scratch and reduce the horror to its bare essentials.
'Oh yeah' said Wilfred soberly. 'I think I read about that'.

(Maupin 1990:161)

HIV prevention work with gay men in Britain, as in the USA, was initially community-based, with gay activists, community organisations and newspapers trying to alert people to the dangers of the new disease. Information in the gay press began to appear in the early 1980s, with Londoners perhaps being best informed through articles in the community newspaper *Capital Gay*. Around this time, new organisations were set up to provide information and support. These usually rose out of the gay community and mainly involved gay men, although lesbians and straight women were involved too. These community-based organisations were set up without any government support; this did not come until much later, despite warnings from doctors and others. In fact, this period has been described as one of widespread government indifference (Watney 1990a; Weeks 1991).

The fact that there seemed to be a strong case for HIV being sexually transmitted meant that much emphasis was put on what came to be termed 'safer sex'. Early safer sex work was influenced by a US booklet produced in 1993 by Berkowitz and Callen entitled *How to have Sex in an Epidemic. One Approach.* This booklet is now widely regarded as the origin of safer sex (Patton 1985; Wagenhauser 1991; Watney 1990b; but see Hart 1993[1]). At the time, there were many disagreements as to the best ways to respond to the disease. Some called for chastity or monogamy, others for less sex or a more selective approach to choosing sexual partners, and there were discussions about not exchanging 'body fluids' (including saliva). In the USA, bitter arguments about closing down public venues which were used for sex divided the gay communities in New York and San Francisco (Foster 1988; Shilts 1987).

Finding ways to encourage people to change their behaviour with little evidence of causation was initially hard. There was apathy, denial, disinterest and resistance to safer sex from some gay men. The activist Larry Kramer is credited by many with forcing US gay men to take note of the disease. This was no easy task. Some of the difficulties in getting messages across are described in his play *The Normal Heart* which was based on his experiences of trying to set up New York's Gay Men's Health Crisis. Most gay organisations in America were initially uninterested. As Foster (1988) notes, gay men had fought against heterosexism and what they saw as restrictive cultural ideas about sex in the 1970s and many saw the move towards safer sex as repressive. It was Larry Kramer's '1,112 and counting' cover story in the *New York Native* that seems to have finally shocked many gay people into action:

> I am angry and frustrated almost beyond the bounds of my skin and bones and body and brain can encompass. My sleep is tormented by nightmares and visions of lost friends and my days are flooded by the tears of funerals and memorial services and seeing my sick friends. How many of us must die before all of we living fight back?
>
> (Kramer 1983:1)

In Britain too, safer sex information and news of 'gay cancer' was not always well received, as Garfield has noted:

> As a rule, liberated gay men didn't like to be told how to live their sex lives; restrictions were seen as an infringement of their hard-won civil rights; it was no longer illegal to have sex between consenting adults over 21, and just let the new moralists – doctors, health educationists, whoever – tell them otherwise.
>
> (Garfield 1994:28–9)

Kowalewski (1988) argues that because sexual activity had an identity-building function for gay men, AIDS challenged the cultural values of gay communities that had centred on sexuality, youth and beauty. It was for this reason that many early writers on the need for safer sex were personally criticised and disliked (Campbell 1989; Gorna 1996).

Some also thought that the disease was just a US problem. Therefore, those with affected friends, lovers or colleagues in the USA felt more concerned and connected to the epidemic, whereas for others safer sex simply became 'don't sleep with Americans' (Garfield 1994:32), something noted by US visitors to Europe at the time (Arning 1996). With time in the UK this changed, with HIV coming to be seen as a disease of the south and Londoners:

> Back in the mid-Eighties my friends in Edinburgh worried about me. For many of them protecting themselves from HIV meant avoiding sex with Englishmen, particularly Londoners. It seemed that the strategy some Londoners had adopted a few years earlier (avoiding sex with Americans) had been recycled

up North. My friends had responded to the information, 'The epidemic has established itself in London' with the strategy 'Don't shag Englishmen'.

(Dockrell 1994:7)

HIV prevention: a community based approach

Initially, most HIV prevention was not developed from health promotion theory but self help.[2] In the USA many men were infected before anyone even realised what the disease was. Thankfully, in the UK the impact was lessened as information did get through, enabling people to change their sexual behaviour and avoid contracting HIV. Knowledge was spread through the commercial gay scene, community organisations, sexual partners and later the media. It is important to note that initially there was a widespread feeling that it was up to gay men and lesbians to alert people to the dangers as no one else would, hence the focus on community based initiatives. The National Network of Lesbian and Gay Switchboards and the emerging voluntary organisation, the Terrence Higgins Trust (THT), played an important role in early information work. With the setting up of the Terrence Higgins Trust in 1982, prevention work became focused on leaflets and roadshows (stalls in commercial gay clubs).

The announcement that HIV was the cause of AIDS in 1984 had a significant impact on health education and enabled the more detailed development of safer sex guidelines. Recommendations related to safer sex developed from the initial calls to cut down on the number of partners and stay in relationships, to having as many partners as were wanted, but having safer sex.

Evidence suggests that many British gay men did change their sexual behaviour in the 1980s (Day *et al.* 1996; Evans *et al.* 1989; Fitzpatrick *et al.* 1989; Hunt *et al.* 1993). The most notable changes were towards greater condom use and less anal sex with casual partners; however, some men also reduced the number of their sexual partners. The levels of behaviour change have been described by Rooney and Scott as 'unprecedented' (1992:5) and by Watney as the 'most effective health education campaign in history' (1990c:13). There is no doubt that some people made remarkable changes to their behaviour. However, there is rarely any evidence put forward to support the enormity of the 'record breaking' claims.

Although much has been made of the impact of early community based work, it is important to remember that levels of prevention work varied across the country. Indeed, in some places little or nothing took place even within gay communities. By the late 1980s, there was evidence to suggest that some gay men had made relatively few changes to their sexual behaviour (Coxon 1988; Fitzpatrick *et al.* 1990; Fitzpatrick *et al.* 1991). This was supported by US research which suggested that behavioural change had been more pronounced among certain groups of gay men (Bailey 1995; Kotarba and Lang 1986). It seems that behaviour change was not as widespread as originally thought.

Government response

In 1985 the government began to give the newly formed THT small sums of money, thereby using it to promote policies which it felt it could not promote directly itself. Weeks (1991) has suggested that government reluctance to become involved was in part fired by their commitment to other policies at the time, including cutting NHS expenditure. Indeed, it is important to recognise that HIV first appeared at a time of reassertion of 'traditional' moral values and the initiation of marketing and managerialism in the new NHS. This had profound effects on reactions to the epidemic:

> The identification of such a health crisis coincided dreadfully with the growth of a moral climate which sought a return to 'traditional values', while attempts were simultaneously being made to transform economic and social policies in the direction of a new individualism and against welfare traditions. This meant that few resources outside those available in the communities at risk were directed at the crisis until the epidemic was almost out of control. As the epidemic spread to other marginal communities and groups, especially the poor, the black and drug users, and barely seemed to touch the 'normal' heterosexual population in most Western countries, even as it was beginning to devastate the poorer countries of the globe, the association of AIDS with the perverse, the marginal, the Other, the disease of the already diseased, gave a colour and stigma to those affected which has persisted, even as community-based organisations, governments, with varying degrees of energy and enthusiasm, and international agencies struggled to contain the spread of infection.
>
> (Weeks 1995:16)

Davies *et al.* (1993) suggest that beyond the projected growth of the epidemic, and concern about the 'spread' of HIV to the heterosexual population, it was media attention and lobbying that finally pushed the government to move. As Bennett and Ferlie (1994) have noted, by the early 1980s community based organisations were beginning to have an impact:

> Nationally and at a local level, social movements and SMOs (social movement organisations) played an important role in the development of the strategic response to HIV/AIDS and were often the first bodies to display concern (from 1982–3 onwards). Not only did they act as direct service providers themselves ... but they also lobbied the statutory sector to move the HIV/AIDS issue further up the 'official' agenda.
>
> (Bennett and Ferlie 1994:97)

This meant that such organisations came to have more of an influence on policy and decision-making (Aggleton *et al.* 1993). However, government policy lagged behind expressed concerns and, despite having been informed by advisors and lobbyists since 1983, there was no action until 1985 when a programme was put in place to check blood supplies and a special advisory group on AIDS established. By 1986, large amounts of money were being set aside for HIV prevention and care and the Terrence Higgins Trust in London received a huge increase in their grant from the government.

The first large scale HIV prevention effort funded by the government did not take place until 1986. It took the form of an information campaign, launched in January 1987, which consisted of leaflets entitled 'Don't Die of Ignorance' which were posted through every door in Britain, and a series of ominous television adverts portraying HIV as a killer sweeping the land. The use of television media was continued in the first World AIDS week in 1987 which showed a variety of HIV related programmes. In this campaign, there was clear evidence of panic about the possibility of a large epidemic and a move towards the message of 'AIDS affects everybody', which highlighted the dangers of the disease for the whole population. Importantly, neither the leaflets nor television adverts specifically addressed gay men; those most affected by the epidemic. Indeed specific government campaigns aimed at gay men did not appear until 1989. It has been argued therefore that for many gay men initial government action came too late and in forms that were inappropriate (*Capital Gay* 1988b; Watney 1989). While this may unfortunately be true, this argument fails to recognise that the initial government campaign was probably inappropriate, with subsequent research suggesting that this work was seriously limited in effectiveness (DHSS/Welsh Office 1987; Homans and Aggleton 1988).

Statutory responses

For a long time, the statutory response continued to lag behind the work of community based groups.[3] In many areas little happened locally until 1989 when the government specifically allocated money for HIV prevention and directed that each district health authority set up local advisory groups. As Bennett and Ferlie (1994) put it, it was individual interest, and in some cases personal ambition, that were often key in terms of moving HIV as an issue forward in the early days. This meant that geographically responses were patchy until government policies, and in some places the numbers of people affected, turned HIV into a local organisational issue.

The statutory sector's delay in responding to HIV meant that voluntary organisations came to be seen as experts and were often able to exert a large influence on policy. This later presented challenges to the statutory sector, especially as many of the former organisations had quite radical roots and a core of personally motivated and passionate workers:

> These were very different organizations from most of those that the statutory sector was used to dealing with. Their membership were neither willing to act as an uncritical voluntary labour force, told what to do by those nominally 'in charge'; nor did they wish to act unilaterally as autonomous organizations. Instead they saw themselves as having a key role to play within the statutory

sector, in preventative activity, in service planning and delivery and in developing policy, and they demanded collaboration and involvement in a quite unprecedented way.

(Bennett and Ferlie 1994:49)

By the late 1980s, however, there were huge numbers of people working in the field, reflecting what has come to be referred to (by some) as the 'AIDS industry' (Gorna 1996; Patton 1990). HIV also began to receive what some felt was a large amount of money. Nationally and internationally, the response to HIV was immense.

Professionalisation and routinisation

One of the consequences of AIDS becoming part of government and statutory sector responses was that it changed the nature of AIDS work. As Patton notes, writing from a US perspective:

The new [AIDS] industry developed a vision of itself and of AIDS work that stood in sharp contrast to the early community activism, in which there were few distinctions between organizers, activists, people living with AIDS, and sympathetic medical workers. It inscribed a rigid role structure which construed 'victims', 'experts' and 'volunteers' as the *dramatis personae* in its story of AIDS.

(Patton 1990:20)

One consequence of this was the expansion of voluntary organisations that began to employ more paid staff. This was a move Patton has called from 'grassroots to business suits', and is described by Bennett and Ferlie (1994:167) as a period of 'consolidation, formalisation and routinisation'. Many voluntary organisations were seen to move away from their roots in gay communities. In some cases, gay men were even moved away from frontline contact with 'the general population' (Schramm-Evans 1990) and organisations tried to promote an image of being accessible to everyone rather than simply gay men (Prout and Deverell 1995; Weeks *et al.* 1994).

In part, these changes may have been linked to maintaining funding, the incorporation of HIV into the large and bureaucratic NHS and the need to appear professional and respectable. This tension between balancing funding principles with those of community based work has long been recognised, and is not unique to HIV (Baker and Craig 1990). At the same time, however, NHS reforms encouraged greater professionalisation by forcing organisations to compete more directly for funds. New funding systems often limited creativity and flexibility, which meant that some organisations became less activist and radical.

During this period HIV also became less of a government and public health priority. In 1993, AIDS lost the special priority status it had been given by the Department of Health. There were many financial implications that followed from this 'downgrading' of HIV. Special ring-fenced budgets that had been set aside for HIV treatment and care were ended as HIV came to be treated like any other disease (Small 1994). There were also large cuts in government grants to major organisations like THT (by now the UK's largest HIV voluntary organisation) and London Lighthouse (a specialist centre for people with AIDS). Lack of media interest, and the fact that the predicted large scale epidemic did not seem to have occurred, created a general belief that too much money was being spent on HIV. In many cases, HIV became incorporated into more generic sexual health work, therefore losing some of its special status.

Re-gaying HIV

With the mainstreaming of HIV, greater involvement of the statutory sector, and growth of voluntary organisations, changes began to occur in both the prevention messages put forward and the groups targeted. For a number of reasons, the balance of work shifted towards more generic work and less work with gay men. With hindsight, it seems that the success of earlier 1980s community-based initiatives led to a situation where the needs of gay men were felt to have been met. The fact that globally heterosexuals were now most at risk also reinforced prevention messages that 'AIDS affects us all'. This period from the mid-1980s onwards has therefore come to be known as the de-gaying of AIDS. As King writes in his book which chronicles this process in Britain:

> 'De-gaying' is the term used to describe the denial or downplaying of the involvement of gay men in the HIV epidemic, even when gay men continue to constitute the group most severely affected, and when the lesbian and gay community continues to play a pioneering role in non-governmental (and sometimes governmental) responses.
>
> (King 1993a:169)

Although it is now generally agreed that a de-gaying of the epidemic did indeed take place in the late 1980s and early 1990s, there is less agreement as to how it happened. De-gaying was a complex process caused by a range of factors. As King (1993a) notes, some of these were unplanned and others were deliberate strategies, at the time carried out in good faith. The main contributory factors seem to have been: early predictions of the direction of the epidemic, based on little information, which overemphasised likely increases in heterosexual transmission; the reporting of national and international statistics, which emphasised the rate of increase amongst heterosexuals rather than the numbers of gay men infected; statutory and government campaigns which pushed 'AIDS affects everybody' messages and neglected the specific needs of gay men; a move by many voluntary organisations away from targeting gay men (who it felt had been reached) to prioritising work with other groups; growing concern not to stigmatise gay men by targeting them alone with prevention messages; and fears of losing funding by concentrating on gay men's work (Gorna 1996; Gorna and Harris 1996; King 1993a; Watney 1990c; Weeks *et al.* 1994).

Several writers have linked the de-gaying of AIDS directly to statutory organisations' involvement in the epidemic, arguing that it was the professionalisation of the field that led to the downplaying of work with gay men and a move away from community based responses (King 1993b, see also Patton 1990):

> The grass-roots activism which had resulted in the precipitous decline in the transmission rate among gay men was allowed to wither and atrophy, as a professionalized model of health education took over, in which promoting safer sex was a job done by workers to 'clients', rather than a strategy of resistance to the epidemic that was shared between gay men and reinforced by peer pressure. Lesbian and gay groups tried not to involve themselves in the epidemic for fear of giving the impression that AIDS was a 'Gay disease', and AIDS organizations which were originally set up by gay men to fight for gay men's interests went into a bureaucratic closet.
>
> (King 1993a:x)

At around the time that issues related to de-gaying were gaining momentum, figures began to appear suggesting there were continuing and increasing levels of unsafe sex among gay men (Hunt *et al.* 1991). Some HIV prevention workers and researchers were concerned that not enough was being done to sustain the changes gay men had made to their sexual behaviour in the early 1980s. In 1991, groups of concerned gay men working in HIV prevention began to meet and discuss how to refocus the epidemic on the needs of those most affected. A major conference held in London in 1991 to highlight the neglect of HIV prevention for gay men by the statutory sector was part of this move to 're-gay' AIDS.

In Britain, one of the most important steps in the re-gaying process was the publication of the results of a national survey of HIV prevention work aimed at gay men (King *et al.* 1992) entitled *HIV Prevention for Gay Men: A Survey of Initiatives in the UK*. This research found an 'alarmingly low level of HIV prevention activity specifically targeting gay and bisexual men, who nevertheless continue to be the group most at risk' (1992:1). This was the case despite the fact that there had already been clear guidance from the Department of Health that work with gay and bisexual men should be made a key priority in all district health authorities. In response to a telephone questionnaire, only 34 per cent of the 226 district health authorities and voluntary organisations surveyed reported having undertaken work with gay and bisexual men. The most common reason given for this lack of work was that staff did not know how to contact gay men. Other reasons included a felt lack of skills to do the work; because there were no gay men locally (as evidenced in the infamous quote: 'We've no homosexual community here, you might try district *[name]* – they have a theatre'); because local prevention work was not targeted; HIV prevention work had been prioritised with other groups; or because it was felt that other organisations were doing this work. This report had an enormous impact on future gay men's work. By highlighting the lack of work taking place, many local health authorities were shamed into beginning work with gay men.

However, there were other factors that put gay men's work back on the agenda. These included new directives from the Department of Health to prioritise work with gay men (DoH 1992, 1993), and a more widespread recognition of the effects of the de-gaying process. In addition, an important influence was the local impact of the national pilot community-based HIV prevention projects for Men who have Sex with Men set up in four cities in the UK, which showed that the statutory sector could successfully support work with this target group. Some of these projects had an impact on neighbouring authorities, which set about funding similar work (BOSS 1994; Prout and Deverell 1995). Indeed, one of these pilot projects went on to become one of the largest gay men's projects in the country working across six health districts.

Efforts to re-gay AIDS were definitely successful. Two years later, when a similar survey of health authorities was undertaken, the authors found evidence of 'a significant increase in the targeting of gay and bisexual men within HIV prevention work' (Anderson *et al.* 1994). Out of the 123 organisations surveyed this time, 86 per cent reported having targeted prevention work with gay and bisexual men in the preceding year, and 49 per cent were now funding specific posts for HIV prevention work with gay men. The range of work undertaken had also broadened, with more specific work on the commercial gay scene and more funding of the voluntary sector. This led the authors to conclude that:

> Work with gay men and bisexual men is now on the agenda of HIV prevention purchasers in almost all health authorities. Where it is not, there is almost always evidence that it soon will be.
>
> (Anderson *et al.* 1994:10)

The importance of work with gay men was reaffirmed at the 1995 launch of *An Evolving Strategy* by the Department of Health's HIV/AIDS Health Promotion Strategy Group. As a newspaper report at the time put it:

> After 13 years of tackling AIDS, the Government has admitted that health and community groups are the best educators in the fight against the HIV epidemic ... the Government is set to target 'high risk groups', such as young gay and bisexual men, in future HIV and AIDS health promotion campaigns.
>
> (Teeman 1995)

This re-gaying of AIDS brought large numbers of new workers into the field. In the early 1990s, there had been very few gay men's workers in the country and outreach work in particular was seen as very new, risky and innovative. By 1994, however, eighty-eight health authorities were funding outreach work on the gay scene and in public sex environments (Anderson *et al.* 1994) in a bid to widen the reach of HIV prevention initiatives and to target safer sex messages. This meant that the outreach work begun in some places in 1990 became well established and workers in these projects were often contacted for advice. By the mid-1990s there were gay men's workers in most districts, regional gay men's workers' forums, training courses, books, conferences and reports all addressing work with gay men. The result of this was to create a more specialised field within HIV prevention that was very well networked and often competitive.

A further important development which occurred during the research was the birth of a new organisation: Gay Men Fighting AIDS (GMFA). The emergence of this group was directly linked to the re-gaying of AIDS. As Scott writes:

> GMFA started because a group of gay men working and volunteering in the HIV field were aghast and angry!!! We were going around like walking exclamation marks!!! It looked like everything that could go wrong in the handling of the epidemic for gay men was going wrong ... . It seemed like there was a multi-million pound AIDS industry, very little of which gave a toss about, or understood gay men. At the same time we could see that there were large numbers of well-meaning individuals who cared a lot but had become trapped in an organisational culture, basically heterosexual and homophobic. A professional bureaucracy had taken over which devalued the skills and experiences of gay men.
>
> (Scott 1993:1)

GMFA was formed by several gay men prominent in the re-gaying of AIDS who had lost faith in the ability of existing organisations to undertake appropriate and effective HIV prevention work for gay men. It was set up solely to work with gay men and saw its primary goal as recreating the same kind of community-level educational activities that had been present at the start of the epidemic (King 1993a; Scott 1993), moving away from what were seen as 'over-professionalised models of education'.

The birth of GMFA was not without criticism (see Gorna 1996 and King 1993a for more detail). Although it is true that very little work with gay men had previously taken place, it was often asserted that no work at all had existed. This understandably angered those who had been involved in HIV prevention work with gay men as they felt their work had been overlooked and neglected (see Miller 1994). Such views were fuelled by the fact that key figures in the re-gaying movement were London-based and felt to be ill informed about work taking place elsewhere in the country. Thus important work by the Aled Richards Trust in Bristol; the first detached outreach work with Men who have Sex with Men in Sheffield; the HEA MESMAC projects (which undertook some of the first targeted work in the UK with black men) and others was frequently overlooked. Indeed, the report by King *et al.* (1992) had shown that one-third of organisations had done some work with gay men (though often this work had been very small scale).

A further criticism was that those involved in the re-gaying movement often seemed to absent themselves from any involvement in the de-gaying process, even though many had been actively involved in AIDS organising for a long time.

Indeed, some HIV workers complained about what they saw as the re-writing of history in order to explain how de-gaying happened (Taylor 1995). Furthermore, concerns were expressed about the reintroduction of a focus on risk groups, and an over-focus on gay men at the expense of other groups (Davies *et al.* 1993; Field 1992; Gorna 1996).

With re-gaying also came assertions that only gay men were able to undertake successful HIV prevention work with gay men and there was discussion of the need for gay only services (Scott 1995a). The role women had played in the early days of community organising was rarely recognised, and those women working with gay men were often made to feel very uncomfortable (Gorna 1996; Deverell and Bell 1993). Issues about who should do the work became the subject of much argument and debate within the field.

New debates

With re-gaying, and an increase in work targeted at gay men, debates within the field shifted towards HIV prevention methods and outcomes:

> Over the past few years, those of us who have campaigned for the re-gaying of AIDS can justly claim that we've secured a much greater level of funding for gay men's safer sex campaigns. Now that the fight for quantity has largely been won, it's high time we focused on quality. We need to confront the question of whether the money is being spent effectively on worthwhile campaigns that are helping to prevent new infections. If not, the money might just as well be left in the health authorities' coffers, and the growing gay men's AIDS sector will amount to little more than jobs for the boys.
>
> (King 1995:8)

In the mid-1990s, greater national attention came to be focused on the effectiveness of safer sex messages and interventions (Hart 1995; Hickson 1995), with intense debates taking place about whether or not HIV prevention works (Scott 1995b; Watney 1995a). These debates linked to wider health service concerns about outcomes, effectiveness and quality and efforts to promote the randomised controlled trial as the 'gold standard' in the evaluation of HIV prevention (Bonell 1996; Clayton 1993; Kingman 1994).

The content of local work also changed to focus more on the complexities of relationships and the role of HIV antibody testing in safer sex (Dockrell 1996; Hickson and Maguire 1996). The diversity of different men's needs was also newly emphasised (*F***sheet* 1999; Prout and Deverell 1995) and there were new calls to include HIV positive men more fully in HIV prevention work (*Positive Nation* 1995; Ward and Jones 1996). The growing sophistication of HIV prevention work, as well as news of advances in treatment, seemed to reflect the fact that the sense of crisis was over.

By the late 1990s, for gay men HIV was becoming endemic rather than epidemic, entailing the need for different kinds of information, support and responses.

There had been a consolidation of organisations as changes in funding caused some smaller organisations to close and larger ones to merge. The work itself had shifted to include more emphasis on detailed, long-term sex messages and more one-to-one counselling and groupwork. In addition, with the launch in 1998 of the Community HIV and AIDS Prevention Strategy (CHAPS) (an England-wide health promotion programme for gay and bisexual men), attempts were made to promote a more strategic and evidence based approach to HIV prevention.

HIV, government and gay men

The relationship between gay men and AIDS is complicated. Several writers have discussed how the development of gay communities in the 1960s and 1970s meant that there was a basis for organised responses to the disease and groups for governments to consult with and recognise (Altman 1988, 1994; Patton 1985). However, it also meant that there were clearly identified targets for scapegoating, as well as routes for the virus to travel along. The association of AIDS with gay men means that for some it has been seen as a disease of choice, self-inflicted by 'gay lifestyles' (Watney 1995a). This has meant that at times AIDS has been seen as a gay rather than a public health issue, something that Altman suggests symbolises the marginalisation of gay men from society (1988). These reactions are built on what Patton (1985) has called the trilogy of 'homophobia, erotophobia and germophobia', and for some AIDS has provided a new space in which to vent their homophobic feelings. The fact that so many out gay men and lesbians are involved in AIDS organising meant that they were an easy target and AIDS organisations have often been attacked for wasting taxpayers' money on promoting homosexuality.

A major issue throughout the history of the epidemic has been the relationship between community-based organisations and government. This relationship has changed over time but has often created profound dilemmas. As Altman has put it in his book *Power and Community:*

> Community organizations need to walk a fine line between seeking to influence the agenda and performance of governments and becoming subsumed into the interests of the state.
>
> (Altman 1994:162)

Voluntary organisations need to engage with the state to secure funds, gain support for their work and trigger organisational change. However, they have often been placed in the position of providing services to communities that governments refuse to acknowledge for fear that they will be accused of 'promoting' either drug use or homosexuality (Watney 1991). Thus, AIDS has profoundly changed the relationship between gay men and governments. As Foster notes:

In those pre-epidemic days the major theme of political action was to get government off our backs. Today, the theme is to make government a partner in solving the research, education, and care and treatment issues raised by the epidemic.

(Foster 1988:216)

Relations between the government and HIV voluntary organisations have often been tense. Indeed some activists have gone so far as to see AIDS as a form of genocide caused by government inaction (Kramer 1990). Delays in government responses and organisational homophobia are not a good basis for building alliances. Indeed, the initial neglect in addressing HIV, and the inappropriateness of many responses has led Watney (1990a) among others to argue that gay men are seen as a 'disposable population', or as one person in this study put it 'not as important as babies'.

One major source of frustration for prevention workers has been the obstructive role that government has exerted over their efforts. Examples of this include the 'toning down' of images and language in prevention messages, as well as censorship through funding. The most visible examples of this can be found in the work of the former Health Education Authority whose actions were, in the early days at least, subject to substantial government interference (Beattie 1991). From the start, HEA campaigns were criticised within the gay press (*Capital Gay* 1988b, 1988c; Burton 1989; *Pink Paper* 1988), at times being described as 'actively harmful' and at other times being the butt of jokes. In 1991, a letter was sent to the All-Parliamentary Group on AIDS criticising the HEA for neglecting gay men and undertaking insufficient and inappropriate work (King 1991). Indeed, an HEA safer sex campaign consisting of factual cards for gay men received a letter from the THT Gay Men's Health Group identifying twenty-six 'blunders'. These criticisms resulted in one card being withdrawn and pulped (*Pink Paper* 1991). The difficult relationship between the HEA, gay community and some HIV organisations came to a head in 1992 when its Men who have Sex with Men advisory group resigned *en masse*, saying they could no longer work with the HEA.

Although there can be no doubt that government interference was often fuelled by homophobia, and a concern not to be seen as promoting homosexuality, the situation is more complicated. As Beattie (1991) has argued, there was a long history of the work of the HEA (later the HEC) being interfered with and suppressed by the government of the day. In 1994, for example, the HEA was forced to withdraw a book about sex for young people after a government minister described it as 'smutty' (*Pink Paper* 1994a). It seems that it is the subject of sex[4] itself that is often the problem (Grey 1993; Holland *et al.* 1990, *Pink Paper* 1994b).

Paradoxically, however, through their opposition to elements of HIV prevention work, governments were forced into detailed discussions about gay men's sexual practices and working with openly gay individuals. Community groups also came to exert some influence over national and local agendas. In Britain, gay men were even congratulated for changing their sexual behaviour by a Conservative government minister in a House of Commons debate on AIDS (Campbell 1989; *Capital Gay* 1989).

While the slowness of organisational reactions to the epidemic understandably caused frustration and disappointment, some activists perhaps had unrealistic expectations and limited understanding of the way large organisations work. In fact, compared to the treatment of some other health issues, the scale of the UK response to HIV disease has been quite impressive. It is too simple to interpret all mismanagement as the direct result of unopposed homophobia (see also Annetts and Thompson 1992).

Working with the statutory sector

In the 1990s, the increase in numbers of paid HIV prevention workers in the statutory sector brought more gay men into the NHS. For many of these, moving from the voluntary to the statutory sector was a frustrating experience as they found their new employment more hierarchical and rule bound. Gay male workers who had been brought in to provide gay community expertise and contacts often found that their daily work entailed dealing with homophobia within their own organisations (Prout and Deverell 1995). Indeed, anyone involved in gay men's work could find themselves having to deal with their colleagues' reactions to this new and controversial work.

More positively, HIV prevention and care forced the statutory sector to deal with out gay men's needs, often for the first time (Griffiths 1995; McNestry and Hartley 1995). In many cases there were significant improvements in both service provision and staff attitudes, though there is little room for complacency.

Gay community, politics and HIV

The HIV field is highly politicised. To some extent, this is related to the nature of the disease for, as Kramer (1990) points out, there is nothing about HIV and AIDS that is not political. However, it also reflects the fact that many HIV workers had a background in gay politics or have been active in gay community organisations. As Watney recalls:

> Looking back, I can see that the degree of my own personal involvement with HIV/AIDS was unusual … it also strikes me how comparatively few of my gay contemporaries got involved in HIV/AIDS work. Those of us who formed the first and second generations of British NGOs (Non Governmental Organisations) came almost without exception from the pre-AIDS gay movement which emerged in the wake of gay liberation.
>
> (Watney 1995b:1)

Gay politics in fact had a substantial impact on HIV prevention. As Altman (1989) and Maclachlan (1992) describe, there are many parallels between HIV work and early gay liberation movements, including the stress on the importance

of positive images, empowerment, self-esteem and building community infra-
structures. At times, this has meant that gay men's HIV work has been criticised by
other gay men for using HIV as a bandwagon for gay rights (Davies *et al.* 1993;
Hickson 1995; Hickson and Keogh 1995) rather than for effective prevention. The
debate is complicated, however, because improving self-esteem and fighting
homophobia can also be seen as essential in the development of an effective HIV
response.[5]

The coming together of gay and HIV politics sometimes creates a heady mix.
There are large numbers of gay men involved in HIV prevention that often share
sexual or social networks. This networking means that gossip, backbiting and
competitiveness are rife and debates are often constructed in ways that are highly
political and emotional. More positively though, these close relationships can lead
to greater collaboration and news travelling quickly through existing networks.

By highlighting important questions about identity, sexuality and community
(Prout and Deverell 1995) HIV disease can be seen to have had a somewhat contradictory effect on gay communities. On the one hand it has raised questions of difference and diversity (Murray 1992) and provoked discussion of community
attachment. On the other hand, HIV can be seen to have strengthened lesbian and
gay communities (Padgug and Oppenheimer 1992:35). Indeed, Altman (1986) and
Plummer (1988) suggest that HIV disease has been a powerful motivating and
organising force. This can be seen in the way that new organisations have been
generated, as well as the emergence of support networks (Meldrum 1993). Both
Altman (1989) and Weeks (1995) have emphasised the ties of friendship and love
that have developed between gay men through the need for safer sex and caring for
those who are ill. Watney (1994) writes that friendship between gay men has been
a crucial source of support, and, for Adam (1992), this caring among gay men has
been the 'silver lining' to the epidemic.

Gay men, identity and lifestyle

'Partners of unknown sero-status' are also known as 'the dating pool'
(Arning 1996:8)

Although not all gay men in Britain have been personally affected by HIV, culturally and symbolically the disease has had a huge effect on many of them. As a
result, for many gay men HIV is now inextricably caught up with their identity.
The changes brought about can be clearly seen (though in a US context) in the
Tales of the City series of novels by Armistead Maupin.

Tales of the City chronicle in a fictionalised form life in San Francisco from the
1970s onwards. There is a noticeable change in tone in the books as the epidemic
hits. AIDS is mentioned for the first time in the fourth book, *Babycakes*, when
the main character Michael (Mouse) Tolliver volunteers for an AIDS Helpline
(Maupin, 1990). In the same book Michael's ex-lover is revealed to have died from
AIDS. The changing nature of gay men's sexual life is portrayed in terms of new
decisions having to be made about where to socialise, and talk of condoms. In

addition, the sense of fear and panic is portrayed in comments about catching HIV from plates. In the final two books, a more serious tone is evident, moving on from tales of sex and parties, to inclusion of the discovery of HIV-related symptoms and trips to doctors.

In becoming part of the common experience of gay men, HIV and AIDS have significantly affected sex and sexual relationships:

> While I am part of the cusp generation of gay men that can remember the time before AIDS, it is requiring greater and greater effort to conjure up the experience of having sex without the spectre of death hovering in the room. Even when you are confident that the sex you are having is as safe as you can make it, the harsh reality of the plague is always present because you know if it were not for AIDS, you would be doing things differently. While all the adverts, shouting variants of 'safe sex is hot sex' are perfectly true and necessary, it is hard to ignore that your sexual repertory has been changed, and that is not by your choice.
>
> (Arning 1996:6)

HIV and AIDS have also greatly impacted upon social and friendship networks. There are differences between gay men of course, but for some the scale of loss has been enormous. It is against this background of diverse needs, fear and support, desire and denial that HIV workers in the health service, in voluntary groups and in the community carry out their work.

Outreach work

Disagreement about the best method of preventing HIV was rife at the start of the epidemic and these debates continue. Outreach work is one way of contacting gay, bisexual and other men who have sex with men, and providing them with information and safer sex supplies. Much outreach work undertaken within HIV prevention follows what Rhodes *et al.* (1991) have defined as a detached outreach model:

> work undertaken outside any agency setting, for example, on the streets, station concourses, in pubs and cafes. This may aim either to effect risk reduction change 'directly' (*in situ*) in the community, or to facilitate change 'indirectly' by attracting individuals into existing treatment and helping services.
>
> (Rhodes *et al.* 1991:3)

There can be many reasons for working in this way; they include: to facilitate needs assessment; to reach people who may have little or no contact with existing groups or organisations; to encourage people to join groups; to get feedback and ideas for new work; and to hand out safer sex resources and information (abridged from Prout and Deverell 1995:71). Regardless of the goals, outreach work involves individuals delivering health promotion messages in locally, and culturally appropriate ways. As such, the main activities involved include:

- preparation (setting guidelines, liaising with the police, seeking legal advice)
- observation and familiarisation (deciding on the best days, times and places to work)
- finding a role (finding ways to fit into the environment, familiarisation with users)
- making contact (deciding who to contact, becoming known, using key contacts)
- giving out information, condoms and lubricants
- making referrals and offering further support
- record keeping (writing up sessions).

Outreach work is often undertaken as part of a wider health promotion strategy, and therefore individual workers may also undertake other activities such as groupwork, advertising or counselling. More recently, outreach projects have begun to put more resources into counselling and providing services on a wider range of health issues than HIV alone in a bid to better address the more complex issues arising when contacting clients.

Outreach sites

Outreach workers work from different bases. Some may use statutory sector offices such as health promotion departments. Others, although employed by the statutory sector, may be housed in their own building. Some work in voluntary organisations, sometimes sharing a building with those undertaking care-based work. Some workers are based in male-only spaces, while others share space with women. However, most outreach work itself occurs in gay pubs, nightclubs and public sex environments. Given that most readers will be familiar with pubs and clubs I will not focus on these here. However, as public sex environments (PSEs) may be less familiar, a brief description seems appropriate.

In the UK public sex environments (PSEs) vary in type and the rules and customs that govern interaction within them (see Bolton *et al.* 1994; Boyz 1995; Hickson *et al.* 1993; Weatherburn *et al.* 1992). The most usual PSEs include cottages (public toilets), cruising grounds (parks, woods, public gardens, lay-bys) and saunas. There is a wide diversity of PSEs, favoured for different reasons and often attracting different types of men. The diversity of sites seems reflected in the variety of men who take part in public sex. For some, cruising is a vital part of gay identity and symbolises a political act against straight society and its rules (Rechy 1978). For others, public sex may be more closely linked to pleasure, danger or the seeking of particular sexual acts (Bartos *et al.* 1993). Consequently, the sexuality of men using these environments also varies.

Sites are busy at different times of the day and year, and change in popularity. Some have a long history of use by gay men, whereas others come and go. One task for outreach workers is therefore to maintain an up to date profile of local PSE sites and their use. It is impossible to give an adequate account of the range of PSEs and the activities that take place within them. However, the following two accounts should provide unfamiliar readers with some idea as to the ways in which PSEs are used.

> I was 14 when I first discovered a cottage. I got cruised by another man in the street in Northampton and we walked to a park and went to a cottage and had sex there … . It made me realise that toilets might have something to do with sex. Then when I moved to London to work I discovered [*names a city centre cottage*] totally by chance.
>
> I remember being totally excited that in the centre of the city's hustle and bustle in the middle of the day there was lots of easy sex to be had. And nobody spoke, it was totally silent. There were two lines of urinals and the glass windows in the cubicles had been blocked out using bits of toilet roll.
>
> All you had to do was stand next to the man you liked the look of and then go into the cubicle for sex. It was sex on tap, there was no cruising, it was instant and honest, and for about six months I went every other day.
>
> (*Pink Paper* 1994c).

10.34 P.M. Greenstone Park.

> NO MOON.
> Jim passes the stone alcove, descends through ashen shadows towards the wall against the trees. He sits on the back of a concrete bench, his outline visible in the mute lamplight. A lean shadow floats by. Attractive, masculine. Jim spreads his legs wide. Two other men are lurking. The lean man – dark, angular, with a gypsy face, the most attractive of the three men Jim has lured – sits next to him on the back of the bench; he too spreads his legs, one knee touching Jim's. Another man squats before Jim. The sexual current rising, the third man bends before the lean one. Rhythmically the two kneeling suck the two sitting, Jim and the man next to him staring at each other … . Car lights flush the area, pulling shadows from the slain darkness. The two separate in opposite directions. The car lights shift. Not the cops – only another hunter driving in.
>
> (Rechy 1978:62–3)

It is important to note that PSEs are structured both spatially and socially (Henriksson and Mansson 1992; Keogh and Holland 1999; Prout and Deverell 1995). Often men will not talk directly to each other, and intentions are signalled in other ways such as through eye contact and body language.

In the UK, all public sex between men is illegal but the policing of PSEs varies. In some areas, the police often find ways to alert users as to when they will be in the area so encouraging men to avoid arrest (Cohen 1992). Other police forces may be more actively involved in arresting and charging people (Jenkins 1990). Outreach projects therefore need to liaise closely with the police. For example, one project worked with the police to clear up used condoms in cruising grounds to stop complaints from the general public (Edwards 1995). The fact that the police often patrol PSEs means that outreach workers often have to find ways to reassure men that they can be trusted and are not there to arrest them.

The extent to which outreach work has now become an accepted part of HIV prevention can be seen in articles in the gay press, as well as in outreach workers appearing in television documentaries (BBC 1996). The early 1990s saw a growth in training courses, guides to doing outreach work, evaluations, needs assessments and reports all addressing the issue (Aggleton *et al.* 1990; Dockrell 1995; Powell and Elkins 1993; Prentice 1994; Sheffield Centre for HIV and Sexual Health 1993, 1996; Stow 1996). This led to a growing occupational confidence, with less anxiety expressed about the work. However, not surprisingly, many outside the field have disapproved of the work. For example, one outreach worker was forced to leave home when information about his job was revealed in the tabloid press (*Pink Paper* 1995b). There have also been several reports of outreach workers, or managers, being attacked or threatened (e.g. Leslie 1993; Mezzone 1996; *Pink Paper* 1994d; *Thud* 1996).

Outreach work received a great deal of media attention in August 1996 following the advertisement of two outreach worker posts in the *Guardian*. Although this type of work had been carried out for at least seven years, the popular press wrote about it as a shocking new development, describing for their readers the 'full horror' of what is entailed.

The *Daily Star*, talked of 'Barmy health bosses' who paid men to 'cruise loos to give safe sex advice to men who meet there for sordid sessions' (Eden 1996), while the *Daily Telegraph* informed readers that 'cruising involves casual buggery' (1996) and called it 'sexual yobbism'. The *Barnet Advertiser* even carried out a phone poll to see if readers agreed with the outreach work. The story was picked up by MPs and, as so many times before, used as a conduit for virulent homophobia. More positively, however, this particular news story led to support for the work being expressed by some MPs and local residents and, importantly, the NHS Health Trust stood by the work.

The symbolic weight of AIDS significantly affects the context within which HIV prevention work is carried out. Importantly, the fears, representations and associations aroused affect reactions both to gay men and to HIV prevention. This means that from within their own organisations outreach workers can experience prejudice or a lack of support, and can feel caught between the needs of the community and the demands of the organisations for which they work. The symbolic nature of HIV and AIDS; the history of the epidemic; the emergence of HIV prevention work from community based responses; the relative newness of HIV prevention outreach; and the context of public sex environments are all important. This background profoundly affects the context within which gay men's HIV prevention outreach work occurs, and shapes the ways in which issues of boundaries and professionalism are experienced.

Part 2

Why boundaries?

Why boundaries are important? Well as I said it's protection of the project, and protection of you as an individual, and protection of the work. Because it would be easy to do something, or say something wrong, or something that the tabloid press would perceive as wrong. You'd see it sort of splashed all over the newspapers, and it would like set gay men's health work back. It might be worse than sort of ten years ago. You know, the sort of moral backlash of health service money being spent on 'these perverts' rather than on sort of newborn babies and hip replacements. I think that['s the] sort of responsibility I feel as a gay man. (Roger, Midlands)

4 Sex, sexuality and work

> At last, it's official. Sex is the ingredient most guaranteed to keep out-trays brimming and productivity rising. A new business morality survey ... reveals that almost a third of office managers would offer someone a job just because they thought they were sexy. Even more shockingly, when asked whether they would promote a staff member for sleeping with them, a significant 13% of respondents said they would. So how can you be sure your employer's been looking at your CV rather than your legs? The truth is you can't.
>
> (Patton 1995:14)

All of the outreach workers in the study felt that sex and work were linked in most occupations and workplaces. For example, work was mentioned as a site of flirting and sexual banter as well as a source of potential sexual partners. However, most felt that this general experience tended to be exaggerated in HIV prevention outreach because of its focus (advice related to sex), the target group (gay, bisexual and other men who have sex with men), and the sites worked in.

For most people, sexuality is not part of their work role, although as Goss and Adam-Smith (1994) point out, it may be tied up in their work identity. The male workers interviewed felt that it was unusual that their sexuality was seen to be so important to their work. A reading of some of the more recent organisational sexuality literature would suggest that this is not the case (see Chapter 1). That said, it is unusual that sexuality is so explicitly defined as a requirement for men, and that it is non-heterosexuality that is sought after in the appointment process. In the following sections I will explore the interconnections between sex, sexuality and work using examples from the interviews to highlight why many workers felt their occupation was unique.

Sex and work

> I think work is quite sexual and everybody knows that. You know, you work at your desk and everyone's seen those pictures of people bending over, their rapt faces are close to each other. But that sort of thing is really true, and

you've got to be very. Well either be lucky and you don't fancy anyone … [or] you've just got to not let it happen, you've got to keep a really tight rein. (Jason, London)

I don't see sex … as separate from work, in the sense that I think that the working environment is a place where people who work together meet and form relationships, including sexual relationships … . I see it [sexuality] as tied to most elements of communication, even if it's in a subtle way. So I do see it as quite linked to the working environment. (Alex, London)

Several outreach workers acknowledged the inter-relationship of work, sex and sexuality and expressed enjoyment that their occupation enabled them to participate more fully in a sexualised work culture, with some saying that they had missed out on this when working in organisations predominantly staffed by heterosexuals (Howard 1995). They spoke about the benefits of having 'a sexual job where you are allowed to be a gay man', being accepted and having the space to explore their feelings and sexuality within work.

Given the sexualised culture of the commercial gay scene, which often crossed into work, the atmosphere in many of the workers' offices itself was very sexual. As Gorna notes, AIDS Service Organisations are often environments 'where gay sex can be an unrelenting feature of conversation' (1996:372). This was confirmed by my participant observation which showed that workers would frequently make comments about other men, and their sexual attractiveness, and walls were often adorned with safer sex posters or other sexualised and explicit imagery. In this way, the work atmosphere parallels in some respects that of other male dominated settings (Cockburn 1983; Jones and Causer 1994; Lippert 1977), with soft porn calendars and sexualised banter, albeit most usually relating to women.

Sexual imagery in the workplace has been the subject of discussion in some AIDS Service Organisations (Cain 1994; Deverell and Prout 1995; Deverell and Rooney 1995). Gorna suggests that it is reflective of a common boundary confusion within AIDS work, when she asks: 'Are these pictures there because gay male workers fancy the models, or to reflect a recent campaign?' (1996:373). Based on the findings from this work, I would suggest they appear for both these reasons, as well as sometimes to display sexuality, encourage male bonding, create a safe space and challenge what are (sometimes) experienced as heterosexist organisational environments.[1] In fact, battles with managers over the display of sexually explicit material were one example given by workers about the homophobic nature of the organisations they worked in.

In common with research from other office and factory settings, the outreach workers in this study would talk to male and female colleagues about relationships, laugh about sex and engage in sexual banter at work. Most found this a pleasurable aspect of work. Interestingly, one of the female outreach workers described how working with gay men had made her into a 'big tart'. As a result, she had started to make objectifying comments and 'sexually harass' men. This offers a new slant to Patton's (1990) observation that gay men give women a licence to talk about sex. It also suggests something of the diversity present in male–female working relationships, which is rarely addressed in the literature.

Both sexual relationships with colleagues, and the use of work as a site to meet sexual partners, are given as examples in the literature on organisational sexuality. A few of the male workers reported having sexual relationships, and fancying or receiving sexual advances from colleagues. For some gay men, work was therefore a potential source of sexual partners; significantly this was not true for the women interviewed. Sex with colleagues was, however, rarely referred to in relation to boundaries; guidelines focused solely on sex with clients and contacts.[2] As Jason said:

> I don't think anybody has ever said you shouldn't have sex with another member of the department, or someone who's a doctor in the GUM [Genito-Urinary Medicine] service, but if it's a sort of a vulnerable member of the public I suppose you're not meant to. (Jason, London)

A few people talked specifically about how their interactions with colleagues were qualitatively different from those with clients. For example, one talked about being very 'po-faced with clients' whereas he swapped 'smutty pictures of men' with the secretaries at work. Such differences have been mentioned in other work. For example Jones and Causer (1994) in a paper on women engineers describe how managers were concerned about the effect of female pin-ups on customers, but not on their female employees. Pictures were therefore only removed from the sites to which customers had access. This difference in relationships between colleagues and with clients is important as it highlights some of the sophistication needed in analyses of organisational sexuality. The fact that there are many different types of sexuality, forms of sexual display and ways of talking about sex in organisations means that much more detailed analysis about who does what, where and with whom is needed.

'Filthy, pervert managers': harassment

> Sexual harassment is likely to occur in most workplaces, across all sectors of employment, in large and in small organisations, according to a survey of employers conducted by the Industrial Relations Services ... . Offences ranged from sexual assault and demands for sexual favours in return for promotion, to leering and derogatory remarks.
>
> (Weston 1992:1)

Much of the literature on sex and work focuses on sexual harassment. Therefore, it is perhaps not surprising that when asked about the relationship between sex, sexuality and work, five people spontaneously talked about sexual harassment from colleagues as an example of how these three issues are linked. All of the cases referred to both by men and women related to experiences in which the harasser was a man.

Research and reported cases of sexual harassment at work have increased rapidly in recent times. Although sexual harassment has been extensively discussed, rarely has it addressed the experiences of men. In part, this is because it is still women who are most likely to be subjected to this behaviour (Coward 1994; *Independent* 1992b). However, this neglect is also a result of sexuality and gender blindness. For example, Brewis and Kerfoot (1994) in a stimulating article on sexual harassment, argue that:

> what is 'bought' in employment is not a sex-neutral ability to perform a service task but the embodied sexuality deemed 'necessary' and appropriate for certain sorts of work. Further, that in so doing, sexuality becomes an intimate part of the workplace. The sexual identity of workers forms an underpinning to the contractual relations between employer and employee.
>
> (Brewis and Kerfoot 1994:10)

They suggest that it is this unspoken aspect of work that leads to sexual harassment:

> Sexuality then may precisely be part of a woman's job, and this may result in sexual harassment. The barmaid for example performs a sexualised role in that she is required to serve her customers with food and drink as well as providing a listening ear, a ready smile and a quick line of backchat to keep the customers amused – in short performs the traditional female role. Hence to sexually harass a barmaid is only to intensify the role for which she has been hired.
>
> (Brewis and Kerfoot 1994:15–16)

Although they use the term 'worker' here, they neglect to say whether their idea of a sexual contract applies to men, and do not describe men being harassed. The fact that Brewis and Kerfoot slip between using terms such as worker and women, sexuality and femininity, suggests that they have a very specific experience in mind.

Where the sexual harassment of men has been discussed (Blundy and Katz 1994; Coward 1994), this is usually in reference to older or more senior women harassing younger men, or as a facet of female dominated workplaces (Patton 1995). Rarely has the issue of harassment between men been addressed, although bullying has been. One important aspect of this research, then, is the way in which men talked about sexual harassment when discussing sex, work and boundaries. For example, Keith described being used as a 'pretty face' by his managers and reported that he was told to go into meetings and flirt in order to secure contracts. He also felt that some of the older gay men he worked with overstepped boundaries of familiarity by making sexual remarks that he found intimidating. He went on to say that some gay male colleagues expressed the attitude that: 'it would be OK for me to talk to you like this in a club, and as we're both gay I can do it in a meeting'. Here, a shared sexuality was seen to override other ways of relating, for instance as colleagues, or as manager and worker. Similar experiences were also reported by two other men who described the actions of gay managers who had harassed them. As Alex reported:

> One of the first things that happened to me in my old job was I was leaning, bending over a filing cabinet to get something out of the bottom drawer and my boss said: 'Oh nice to see you in the appropriate position'. It was like my third day at work or something and I had to actually stop and think about what he'd said and sort of say, no that's not a joke. It might be a joke to somebody I'd worked with for a year and they knew I felt comfortable with, whatever, but I actually had to say something. (Alex, London)

However, harassment did not only come from managers. For example, Jason discussed receiving unwelcome attention from colleagues within his organisation because of his, and his teams', looks:

> You know people fancied us a lot ... and we got that kind of even from colleagues at work who would say: 'You're really dishy'. You know we'd go for a meeting and get patronising comments ... 'They've really employed you for your looks haven't they?' We used to get that loads of times, [I] said 'I hope not'. (Jason, London)

He was frustrated by this patronising attitude which he felt meant that he was not taken seriously at work. Such incidents were distinguished from general sexual banter or flirting, which was felt to be acceptable. Importantly, sexual remarks from colleagues and managers were seen to be different to sexual comments from clients or contacts; the latter were still frequently described as annoying but were tolerated because they were seen to 'come with the job'. In this respect, the workers' experiences are not dissimilar to those reported by female workers in service industries.

Sex and work in HIV prevention outreach

While the outreach workers interviewed acknowledged a general link of sex and work, more striking was the way in which sex and sexuality were viewed as integral components of outreach work. The two were 'impossible to separate'. As Craig put it:

> Well in the type of work we do, then it's not separate at all, in any way is it really? I mean 'cos we're working with people in that sort of arena aren't we? Um ... [the] sex arena and sexuality arena, so it's very difficult to separate that. And also because we're employed because we have a particular sexuality ... in terms of that, then obviously it is part of our work. (Craig, Midlands)

> For my work they're not different, they can't be different. I work in a lesbian, gay bisexual centre, and I work with gay and bisexual men, and part of my role is advocacy around those identities … .And I'm employed because I am a bisexual man, so it is integral to my work. (Mike, London)

Personally, through my involvement in HIV work, I have experienced many of these linkages myself. Undertaking HIV prevention work seems (inevitably) to bring with it connotations of sex and sexual availability. To a degree it is like any occupation, certain questions go with the job. Doctors may be asked about symptoms and treatments, I would be asked about such things as HIV tests, condoms, HIV prevalence figures, cures, causes, gay men's sexual relationships, sexual problems and whether I knew anyone with AIDS. Significantly, though, the content of the work often led to the sexualisation of interactions. For example, when conducting outreach with heterosexual men, handing out condoms would frequently be interpreted as a sign of sexual interest on my part, or would be used as an opportunity for sexual innuendo such as: 'Can I try it out with you?', 'Is that an offer?' and I would get asked for my phone number. Furthermore, when carrying out participant observation on a safer sex stall, which involved young heterosexual men practising putting condoms on dildos, every response on the evaluation questionnaires answering the question: 'What did you like most about the THT Roadshow?' related to myself and the female colleague who had staffed the stall. HIV-related work gives people a licence to talk about sex and workers' ability to discuss sex often seems to be regarded as a sign of sexual availability. As Jason and Nick explained:

> Some people think that because you're out there handing out condoms then you're public property and they can put their hands and their mouths and whatever else wherever they like and that does become very annoying. (Jason, London)

> Because we talk to people about sex, that makes them feel we're sexually available … . So I think that makes the passes that they make at us stronger … . I've had like huge amounts of passes and inappropriate physical contact or whatever. (Nick, London)

Another worker, Rob suggested that an ability to talk about sex communicated an idea that workers 'will be that free with their body'. He described the following experience of four men making sexual advances towards him when undertaking interviews for a needs assessment:

> To them, it's like a really big thing having a young gay man go there and spend some time with them, to talk about being gay, talk about sex … . There were offers of dinner and oh, you know, 'Do have a sherry', all this stuff … . One chap as soon as I got out the car said: 'My what a big strapping lad you are', and then throughout … two hours of interviewing, every question … about

sex or safer sexual practice, what have you, his answer was: 'If I was having sex with you I would' ... . Another chap ... said: 'Oh I've got to go upstairs, I think there's something that might interest you'. And he's an academic, and I thought he might have, you know, some research or something which would be interesting. He came downstairs and hanging out of his flies was this nine-inch dildo! ... I was like *(shriek)*: 'Oh my God'. (Rob, North)

The sexual content of their work, the target group worked with, and the perceived importance of their own sexuality, were some of the reasons given why HIV outreach work implied a close association with sex and sexuality. As Keith (North) put it, 'Sex was on the agenda all the time'. And as Andrew and Tim explained:

> We're a sex project, so sex is the end result of most of what we're talking about. And we work in a highly sexually charged environment and that a day doesn't go by when like 80% of the conversations we have in the office are about sex. (Andrew, North)

> Well you're obviously working with a community of sexual desire as much as anything else ... . It's not the only thing, but I think it's one of the key defining qualities of the gay community, that it's a community of ... pooled and persecuted sexual desire. And you're talking to them about sex, you're not talking to them obviously about heart health, or chiropody, or any of that stuff ... . (So) in all the work that we do we use a kind of language or currency that's sexualised. (Tim, London)

The unusualness of HIV-related work was often commented on, sometimes in a self-mocking way. Workers suggested that as their jobs were unusual, this made the experience of sex and sexuality within work very different:

> You know one day I spent a whole day going through porn magazines to find like the right images, and to get sort of like, you know, the right kind of mood for like a campaign, for a poster we were doing. And it's like, I'm being paid by the Department of Health ... to sit in a room and look through porn magazines, and *(sniggers)* ... that's work! (Keith, North)

As Keith expressed it, people would not normally be paid for carrying out such activities. In fact, for most people reading pornography would probably be regarded as a leisure activity. This serves to underline how the content of HIV prevention work can lead to a blurring of boundaries.

Interviewees often contrasted their experience of HIV work with other occupations, highlighting how HIV was a 'special case'. The difference for those involved in sexual health work was that sexuality was associated with their occupation, not just with themselves:

I don't think it [sexuality] comes up so much in other kinds of work ... . It probably doesn't come up in a post office or, it might do for individuals, but not as a whole I wouldn't have thought. (Sandi, East)

Sexuality as a qualification

For many gay and bisexual male outreach workers, the relevance of their own sexuality to the work had been specified in their job description. This led several to say that it was impossible to divorce sexuality from the work itself:

I don't think it can be separate from this work, because if it wasn't for my sexual identity I wouldn't be doing the work. (Toby, North)

As many perceived their sexuality to be the basis for their employment it is not surprising that their sexual(ity) experiences were seen as primary and integral to the work:

I was employed on the basis that I am bisexual identified, or that I'm gay or bisexual identified. So I use the experience I've had of coming to have that identity ... as an integral part of how I go about my work and how I relate to our users ... . So that's an emotional thing, and that's about an understanding of the people we're working with, their needs. I also use a political understanding I've gained from having that identity, in terms of the advocacy work that we do, and the need to create political change to do a lot of the work that we do. (Nick, London)

K: So do you think you use your own sexuality in doing the work?

I suppose you do, and I think that you have to. Um, I think for one thing that, you have to have shared the same experiences, and know what motivates people to be there [in a PSE/club] in a social situation ... . You are actually able to know what you are talking about, and then that can be identified. (Bill, Midlands)

It is interesting that Bill emphasises the need for knowledge and experience to be identified by others. Some workers felt that it was easier for a gay or bisexual man to signify to a contact that they had the appropriate knowledge, than it would be for a woman. For this reason, gay men were often felt to be the best candidates for this work.

The employment of people with certain characteristics is not uncommon. This is especially the case in service industries and people work, where it has been shown that sexuality and attractiveness are often used as part of a 'sexual sell'. For example, Abraham (1994) in a study of lingerie selling in a department store, noted that all the workers were required by the company to be women. In addition, women's sexuality has been used to secure favours or drum up business. Sexualised advertising using pictures of scantily clad women alongside suggestive captions is a case in point (Jeffreys 1996; Hochschild 1983).

Sexual skills

Outreach workers described several ways in which they were able to use their sexuality within work. A sexualised sell in the form of cruising skills could, for example, be used to make contact with potential service users:

> *K:* And do you think you use your own sexuality in work?

> Uh yeah. I think I do. Like outreach work in cruising areas, sort of identifying who to contact and who not to contact is almost like a process of picking somebody up in the first place. Like you sort of get the vibes from them ... you split the wheat from the chaff. So I suppose that is using ... sexuality as the sort of main tool. (Richard, Midlands)

Using such sexual techniques was seen as vital in gaining men's interest. Workers would try to harness the sexualised atmosphere in the places that they worked to make contact and build rapport. For example:

> What are the first tools that you're using in order to make contact with them [service users]? Well invariably it's body language and for that short period of time you're actually ... using body language in that kind of, I could be a potential lover in their lives. (Erkan, London)

> To work in a, in an outreach field of working with men who have sex with men, you display your body as a sexual being ... you make contact with them, 'cos they like you, or they fancy you, or something like that. Especially in the work I have done in the sauna, because you are half-naked anyway. I mean the only thing that's round you is a towel, it doesn't leave much to the imagination! (Sanjay, Midlands)

Such quotes highlight how sexual interest is used to generate contact, and offer a clear example of the use of the body in work. While not everyone used their sexuality in so direct a way, nearly all felt that cruising skills were important to their work. In fact, the perceived need to use these skills meant that many of the workers felt that only certain people were qualified to do outreach:

> With like streetwork so much of it revolves around pretending to be sexual ... . You're playing the game, you're cruising ... . The reason you can do it is because you've done it in your own life and you're calling on techniques you use. I mean you couldn't just place anyone out there [and] sort of like [say] 'cruise' ... people just wouldn't know what to do, or how to react, or what the little rules are when someone like wanders past, or how much eye contact, how much not, and all that. (Andrew, North)

For some, however, cruising skills had to be acquired for work:

> *K:*   Is that [cruising] something you think you can learn or?
>
> I think it is something you can learn. I can do it better now than I ever used to be able to, but I still can't do it very well. I still get embarrassed and want to giggle and look down and it still feels a bit silly to me you know. (Sean, North)
>
> *K:*   So was it easy to sort of learn all that stuff or?
>
> It was fun to learn yeah. And for us to decide how I was going to dress so that I was quite neutral, I wasn't actually signalling that I was into anything in particular. Um and lots of people don't signal what they're into, so I just had a way of me dressing that, I was mainly open to suggestions, which allowed me to talk to quite a few people. (Sandi, East)

Because sexuality and bodily appearance were used to make contact, workers had to be very conscious of the image that they presented, especially as they did not want to put off potential contacts:

> Particularly amongst like young, gay men then you have to look good, do you know what I mean? So you are always aware of that. You feel like you're sort of being judged on your physical appearance, as much as on your attitude to the work .... People will be more inclined to speak to you if you are young and handsome and trendy and, do you know what I mean? If you are more approachable. And that's a real issue I think ... it has an effect on you as a person. If you don't feel very attractive it's very hard .... You feel as if you are put on the spot somehow and you are being found lacking. (Sean, North)

Interestingly, the pressures created by working in a community that places such emphasis on appearance were rarely seen as a problem by male workers.

Sexuality and trust

Sexuality was also used to gain trust. Several workers reported that they were asked what their sexuality was, which suggested that this information was important.

> And quite often people do ask a lot about my sexuality ... quite often they've had really outrageously bombastic questions like: 'You must be a lesbian', or you know: 'Have you got a girlfriend? What do you do with your girlfriend in bed?', all those sorts of questions which I think are quite outrageous. (Sarah, London)

In terms of building trust, those involved in outreach work with drug users felt that their personal experiences of both drug using and gay cultures were important. As Rachel explained:

I s'pose there's sort of two aspects to that, there's the drug taking aspect, which is often far more pertinent obviously, because we're a drugs project. But by being able to have that background knowledge of the [gay] scene, so people talking to you ... know that you really understand the need that they have to belong to that culture, especially if they're stuck in the bloody closet at work during the week ... . Being able to talk about their problem not being in isolation, you know: 'I know other gay men to whom this has happened, this is a common phenomenon amongst people we see'. That kind of thing makes it really useful. (Rachel, London)

Having the knowledge and experience with which to relate to people's experiences was seen to be vital. To be seen as credible and to gain trust, workers often drew on their own personal experiences. However, which experiences were used depended on the content of the work. For example, all of the Asian and African-Caribbean outreach workers pointed to the importance of understanding the links between sexuality and race.

Although everyone felt they used their personal experiences in some way at work, several people mentioned that this was not always appropriate. Indeed, there were different contexts within which they would reveal personal information or display their sexuality. The use of sexual skills was related both to the context and the content of the interaction. As Nick put it:

I've had to learn through experience ... about how I disclose my sexuality, sexual identity. How I do, when I do and when I don't ... things like liaising with the police and being an out bisexual man, I've learned huge amounts of techniques about how I present myself to the police and what effect that has. (Nick, London)

Workers felt that revealing their sexuality did not always lead to a positive reaction and so they had to judge carefully when and where it was appropriate to employ sexual skills.

As well as using personal experiences linked to their sexuality, workers also drew upon personal experiences of sex. Some even purposefully tried out new techniques in their own sex lives to provide experiences that could be drawn on for work. A few workers reported reflecting on their own experiences in order to think more carefully about the work and how clients might feel. This empathetic approach was felt to make interactions less impersonal and more tailored to the individual. In this way, the worker's private self was brought to work to make it easier to build rapport with clients:

If you're not able to, to look at your own sex life and talk about it ... how can you expect someone else to really? It's like sexuality you know ... unless you've explored it to some extent ... I don't think people are going to be comfortable exploring it with you. (Jill, South)

And being prepared to be honest, I mean like in the groups we work with, and on the [gay] scene as well, when people ask you about what you do sexually ... . You're asking people what they do a lot of the time and you've got to be prepared to say [what you do]. (Andrew, North)

Using personal experiences of sex and sexuality was an important part of how workers related to other men, gained credibility and showed solidarity. Having a shared sexuality with clients could thus enrich work enormously, but meant there was always potential for boundary confusion:

You know that problem of not over-identifying with your clients? [It's] Totally different when you're working with young gay men, because you've been through it ... I felt so happy to be doing the work sometimes, so happy to be just feeling instinctively what people said to me. Instead of having to search for those little identifications, you know, I actually felt them. I'm sure that that confused the boundaries a little bit and made me more of a befriender sometimes, rather than a neutral counsellor. (Erkan, London)

Some men identified very strongly with the client group and for this reason it was suggested that too much emphasis could be put on linking sexuality and sex with work. The work could become overpersonalised, and bringing personal agendas into work so directly could cause complications.

Sex on premises: working in sexual sites

One obvious link between sex and work arises when sex takes place on work premises. While no worker reported having sex in their office, a few did report that they sometimes used places in which they worked as social and sexual sites, even when this was explicitly forbidden by their guidelines. This was particularly the case for those working and living in small towns.

Some workers told me that (named) colleagues had had sex whilst working in clubs or sex venues. However, this was much frowned upon (by management as well) and the ways in which it was talked about suggested it did not happen often. Interestingly, sexual liaisons at conferences were seen to be fine, and widely gossiped about, presumably as these encounters were with colleagues rather than (potential) clients.

Outreach work in saunas, clubs, pubs or public toilets brought workers into contexts where other people were socialising and having sex, and often they had to pass as though they were doing the same, at least for some of the time:

The difference with cruise work is that you are always automatically seen as a cruiser ... . The only men who are on cruising sites at 2 o'clock in the morning are men wanting sex with other men. So, if you start from that premise ... unless you've got neon lights saying who you are, and why you're there, the first premise is that you are there to have sex. (Derek, London)

In these kinds of situation, workers suggested that they needed focus and discipline, as their role was not always easy to communicate:

> Our first point of contact with men is cruising, sexual contact. It's not talking … . It definitely is on a sexual level that you first communicate, um so I think that makes boundaries a very difficult issue, because you're communicating on one level, and then very quickly have to assert where that stops. (Nick, London)

> If you're in an office, you're not there to have sex. If you're in the pub, in a club, you could be there socialising and not there to necessarily tap off. If you're down the [PSE], you're there for sex generally, most of the time, and people are generally isolated and very cruisey, and the only way to establish contact is to cruise … . So you're giving a mixed message, you cruise them then you say: 'Hang on, this is what I am, this is what I'm doing here'. (Sean, North)

The nature of such sites meant that workers had few of the external markers others have to indicate they are at work. They were not in an office but talking about sex in places where people meet to have sex:

> You are in a context where people go to tap off with each other, and have fun and be drunk and things like this. Whereas if you're in an office, you're not in that context, do you see what I mean? So, it's like the atmosphere there is completely different. (Sean, North)

> In outreach, it's really difficult because the boundaries are really invisible. You don't have a building around you to kind of say: 'Once through this door you're entering another organisation, you're entering another set of rules'. You're on territory that is at best, from my point of view neutral, in my weakest of moments I was thinking: 'Well actually this is their territory'. (Erkan, London)

The sexual potential of much outreach work meant that workers had to manage their own and others' sexual feelings. The possibility for sex to happen was felt to be 'much more immediate' than in other occupations:

> And we're in a situation where we meet a lot of people, and we meet them and we talk about sex, and we offer support around sex, and we offer the resources to practise sex. So you, you get to meet more people on a level where that might lead to sex … compared to if I was a train driver. (Nick, London)

Boundaries were thus important in helping to create a work atmosphere in places that for others were constructed as sexual or social. They helped to define activities as work and kept a focus on the task of outreach. In this way, sexual boundaries were sometimes likened to other issues, such as not taking lots of personal phone calls at work. Maintaining boundaries was seen as a form of discipline that enabled a separation of work and personal life, and ensured that work tasks were prioritised:

> You shouldn't mix business with pleasure ... because it ruins your work, ruins your work practice, you become slack at your work. You go with the intention to do that kind of thing [have sex], you don't go with the intention of doing work. (Sanjay, Midlands)

> For paid workers you cannot be having sex while you are working, while you are being paid to work. Um [it's] simple, because you're not paid to have sex, you are paid to pass information, to pass condoms. (Derek, London)

The issue of whether or not to have sex whilst working, or to use workplaces for sex, was discussed fervently with the launch of GMFA's Heath Project (Dockrell 1993; Fisher 1996). This initiative used volunteers to conduct outreach work in cruising sites and allowed volunteers to have sex in their tea breaks. Many workers in the field felt that the voluntary aspect of the work made this acceptable. However, others still found problems with this way of working, for ethical or other reasons (see Chapter 7). Interestingly, GMFA used this work as an example of their strength as a community based project, comparing this to workers in the statutory sector whom they saw as hampered by bureaucratic rules.

Defining relationship with users

The fact that work took place in sexualised spaces made it important to find ways to communicate sexual boundaries. Workers had to find ways to explain their role to service users so that they understood what to expect:

> A good thing about the boundaries is that I was consistent enough to say: 'No I'm here for this purpose', and that must've given them some kind of safety, so that they could go overboard on the flirting, knowing that nothing could happen at the end of the day and that was cool. (Erkan, London)

> Partly because it empowers the people that you are talking to .... It's saying to them: 'I'm not going to try and pick you up, this is not why I'm talking to you', so it clears that kind of out of the way. Because there's always this tension between gay men when you go up and to talk to gay men that: 'Oh he's trying to pick me up', and either they want you to or don't want you to, and that can have an effect on how they hear you.

> *K:*   There's some sort of sexual expectation that has to be resolved?

> There'll be some sexual expectation that's right. And to resolve that immediately is always very good for them as well as for us, because it means that then

they can start to communicate with you on a different kind of level. So they don't have to flirt with you outrageously, or they don't have to ignore you because you're being a pest. So I mean I think that's really important. (Sean, North)

Here, the importance of the boundary was related to the working relationship. Part of the client empowerment workers talked about was seen to work through enabling people to talk about sex without worrying that this would be seen as seductive or lead to a sexual advance. This is a reason other professionals have given for the importance of boundaries (Pope 1989). Indeed, interviewees stressed that because service users may be seeking support or advice on issues related to sex, sexuality or sexual problems, preserving the sexual boundary was crucial. This was because having intimate knowledge about people's sexual practices was felt by workers to put them in a powerful position, for example, potentially they could blackmail clients. Boundaries were thus perceived as a method of ensuring that workers did not abuse their power and that they were taken seriously by contacts:

We're all generally coming from the same point of view, that we realise that as sexual health workers, as employed people, people who have a, you know, a job description to uphold, people who are working in places where people are having sex, or arranging it. That [we're] there as workers, that we have power, and that there's this difference in power. And of course if someone gives you quite personal information, then of course that increases your potential hold over them ... . In which case it's widely accepted that sexual relations are no go. (Rob, North)

In the literature on sexual boundaries in counselling and trusting relationships, having sex with clients is not only described as unethical but also as a form of abuse because it destroys a trusting relationship (O'Gabbard 1989; Rutter 1991). None of the workers explicitly highlighted the prevention of abuse as a reason for drawing boundaries while I spoke to them, but many would probably agree with this idea. Certainly many talked about the need to recognise that power relation-ship between workers and clients was an unequal one. As Tim put it:

Boundaries are what you're offering to people as well, I think that's the other thing ... . If you're working with somebody who has real low self esteem and tries to compensate for that by having lots of men, and you're saying to him: 'No I really like you, and I just think you're fine, and I'm not going to have sex with you'. That's not just about your workplace demands that, that's actually good for him. To hear somebody saying: 'No it's you actually that I like, and we're not going to have sex and you can still get something from this relation-ship' ... . That's not just a boundary preventing something. It's actually the boundary enabling something quite important to go on. (Tim, London)

In this way boundaries were sometimes seen as enabling a special kind of relationship to develop, in which sexual issues could be discussed in a supportive manner. Usually, workers talked about counselling rather than trusting relationships, but they still seemed to distinguish this type of 'professional' relationship from the more informal contact they had with other men:

> I mean obviously if people have got identifiable problems, however good looking they are it's just a realisation in that worker's mind that going to bed with them is probably the worst thing you could do for them.

> *K:*   And why would that be?

> Because it's just a breach of your position. I mean, you can't sort somebody else's problem out whilst they're being emotionally attached to you, whilst they are becoming physically and emotionally dependent on you. That's just not on. (Edward, North)

In this way, workers talked about needing boundaries to communicate the limits of their role and relationships:

> A good example is a guy who's a volunteer at the moment, who apparently is very like together, very sorted, is quite happy about talking to us. And suddenly behind all this there came out all this shit, about he felt he didn't have any friends, he was very isolated, he found it difficult to meet friends on the scene. He's got arthritis and so finds, you know, moving very difficult. Sometimes he's stuck in his flat and he hasn't got any money 'cos he's on the dole. So he hasn't got a phone, he hasn't got access to communications, transport. And then he started talking about how he feels suicidal sometimes, and how he doesn't practise safer sex … . To me, the first thing that signals for me is boundaries, in terms of how I relate to that person. Am I creating a false sense of friendship which isn't there on my part? … . Where their expectations of me are beyond what I am prepared to meet and therefore that is going to damage that individual? (Nick, London)

It is important to note that boundaries here are constructed around the needs of the worker, although with good intention. Thus, although there is talk of empowering the client, it is workers who set the frame of interaction.

> *K:*   Can you say something about how you think clients react to the idea of boundaries?

> Yeah. Well I don't think they care about them. I mean why should they? It's not their business, nothing to do with them really … . If they want to have sex with you and you say: 'Well it's a job and I can't have sex with you', they think it's an excuse. But I don't care particularly … I think some people really get it, some people who might work in a position where they

have boundaries of their own. I think some people really don't understand it. I think some people see the benefit of it as time goes on. (Tim, London)

While maintaining boundaries was seen largely as the workers' responsibility, sometimes it was aided by clients or users themselves. For example, some men reported that not having sex for ethical reasons was often made easier by the fact that they were often assumed to be HIV positive and so seen as sexually taboo. This meant that workers could be put out of bounds by clients too, highlighting the interactive nature of boundary making, which will be discussed further in Chapter 6.

Challenging in organisational contexts

A very different way in which workers used their sexuality lay in their attempts to challenge homophobia at work, and to raise organisational issues related to sexuality. Sometimes this was done as a conscious choice, and at other times because they felt they had little choice other than to do it. For example, some workers described how being open about their sexuality at work meant that it became a way of educating others:

Some people may be frightened of the fact that [you are gay], or [have] never met somebody who's gay, whether that be male or female. And working with them you can actually turn them around … . If you're an out gay person I think you do this all the time. (Sandi, East)

Well you're constantly out all the time, there's no two ways about it, you're out … I mean that's a thing where there's like no boundary between the personal and the professional … . And that I find very useful. I think it challenges people's perceptions about what gay men are … . Because people have said, you know: 'Oh I would never have thought you were gay', professionals: 'I wouldn't have thought you were gay'. (Sean, North)

Interestingly, several respondents reported integrating their sexuality into their work as a way of advocating social and political change and breaking down barriers. This was particularly the case for those involved in community development work where there were explicit aims about changing organisations and promoting equality (see McNestry and Hartley 1995; Prout and Deverell 1995). Work was here seen as a place to campaign and raise awareness around sexuality. Jill suggested that because some gay men have had their sexuality validated through doing HIV-related work; they have begun to use work as a site for sexual politics battles:

HIV is a place where a lot of gay men find a bit of power, find a bit of voice … where what they say matters because they're gay men. Because a lot [of things] can be addressed through HIV. (Jill, South)

Indeed, a few workers said they deliberately used this type of strategy to make some of their heterosexual colleagues feel uneasy:

> I might also use it [sexuality] to guilt trip people, if I want to get something that I really feel should be going on. I don't do that very often, and I think it's a last resort, but it is a mechanism I will use. (Nick, London)

Some gay men were very aware of the power they had within 'equal opportunities culture', and used their sexuality to gain support by appealing to 'liberal middle class feeling'. Others said they sometimes flirted to get what they wanted. In this way individuals or organisations could be embarrassed into providing services or resources for gay men. However, others reported a down side to being openly gay or bisexual at work. The fact that they had been employed *because* of their sexuality, rather than that they were doing a job and happened to be gay or bisexual, was an issue that could cause problems. A major factor here was that their occupation immediately made their sexuality public:

> Going into meetings and going [into] ... forums where, you know, where you're maybe feeling a bit vulnerable, or powerless, or intimidated or threatened and you [are] ... automatically and instantly, you know, identified as a gay man. So your sexuality is ... up for open debate ... and comment as well ... . Sometimes that is a real strain. (Keith, North)

> I think all the work, at all levels really, it's about being very public about our sex and our sex lives, and I mean also about our sexuality. You know, I can't tell people what I do without them knowing I'm a gay man, or assuming that I'm a gay man. (George, North)

This meant the workers' job titles made public something usually regarded as private.[3] For workers, the instant identification of their sexuality could lead to being in the front line of homophobia or prejudice:

> We take the flak far more than maybe your general gay man does. Or, you know we come into direct firing line if you like, with people ringing us up with obscene phone calls, and like all the [negative] attitudes at social services and the education department. (Sean, North)

The visibility of the workers' sexuality also affected how colleagues at work perceived them. For example, they could be assumed to be pursuing a vested interest as 'a professional gay man'. In this way, legitimate demands could end up being viewed as special pleading. Or individuals might be accused of bringing personal agendas into work. This meant that workers could find themselves in the double bind of having been employed because of their sexuality, but being criticised for being 'over-involved' if they tried to raise issues related to homosexuality at work.

Own sexuality

Another reason given for the need for sexual boundaries was to manage occasions where workers or clients (or both) wanted to have sex with each other. This was recognised by one gay worker who jokingly noted that it might help in drawing boundaries 'If we were all straight!' This raises an important point. As a straight woman worker put it:

> If I was working with this many men that I work with, but they were all straight, I imagine I'd spend a bit more time thinking about it [sex] *(laughs)*. But as it is … most men I meet through work I assume they're gay until proven otherwise you know *(laughs)*. So, I just never really think about it [sex]. (Jill, South)

Carrying out counselling or giving out safer sex advice and condoms could be made difficult where workers felt sexually attracted to contacts or clients. Although this was accepted as inevitable, it was sometimes still difficult to handle:

> You see people you fancy, and it does make it quite hard to talk to [them]. It's harder to talk to somebody you fancy the bollocks off. Much harder. (Sean, North)

> Being a gay man makes it difficult very much I think … . Like the culture of like sex between gay men, and that currency I suppose. That can make it very difficult to keep those boundaries. Especially if a man is really good-looking or very attractive or whatever … and is sort of like he's coming on to you, I mean it's massively difficult. (George, North)

> In one case I actually had to just leave, I just left. And I was actually quite upset about it because I really wanted to, to have sex with this guy … But I was working in that set time. And it's like; 'Well if I did it no one would know'. And I thought 'But you would know, and you know that you shouldn't', and its like that's why. Because I didn't even want it to get to that stage. (Isaac, Midlands)

Although workers occasionally felt attracted to clients, it was usually turning down sexual advances which was seen as the main focus for boundaries:

> The boundaries most people have to manage isn't wanting to have sex with men that they're working with and telling them they can't. The real boundary most people have to deal with is men wanting to have sex with them and them saying 'No'. That's the reality. (Tim, London)

As workers became known, service users began to realise what their role entailed. However, some service users continued to press workers for sex. For this reason, boundary making became a continuous and complex process.

Conclusions

Sociologists have traditionally written about sex and work as though they are separate areas of life. This view does not fit the experience of the outreach workers interviewed here for many of whom sex, sexuality and work are complexly intertwined. How separate sex and work were seen to be depended on what people felt work was about and how they perceived their role. Most workers felt that flirting and using 'sexual energy' within their work was acceptable. However, they argued that it was inappropriate to act on sexual feelings whilst working. This meant they had to find a way to balance their use of sexual skills with maintaining personal and professional boundaries.

Most of the workers were more specific about the ways in which sex and sexuality were linked to work, and had developed clear ideas about the need to keep them separate:

> I really believe that for a whole range of reasons, some of them maybe more practical actually than ethical or moral, having sex and work, doing your work, should be separate. Even if the content of your work is to do with supporting safer sexual behaviour. But I don't think that's necessarily true of sexuality. Obviously sexuality has a real part to play in the workplace. (Tim, London)

> Would you expect any other person in the health promotion or health framework … to have sex with their clients … . If you went along to your GP and you said 'Well I'm having [sexual] problems', you wouldn't expect your GP to say 'Well I'll show you how to do it' … . To be frank yes, be explicit in what you're talking about, and not being bashful yes. But to actually have sex with people is a completely different thing. (Bill, Midlands)

For this reason, the relationship of sex to work was felt to be very different to that of work and sexuality. Workers felt that their own sexuality, and issues related to sexuality, was inseparable from work, whereas for many having sex should be kept separate from the work they did.

5 The impact of work on personal life

In Britain, there is a strong cultural imperative to maintain a social life space separate from that of paid employment. 'What are you doing at the weekend?' and 'What do you do after work?' are well-used questions. For outreach workers living and working in the same community, it was often difficult to maintain such clear boundaries between places of work and personal life. Because so many outreach workers were themselves gay or bisexual, this meant that their places of work were very often also places of socialisation or areas in which they met sexual partners. Outreach work was not like that of other occupations:

> I think that the issue of gay men working with gay men has never really been broached before. I mean, we socialise with our client group because we're gay men, and we go out on the scene with the people we work with – unlike social workers who don't go out with their clients, they don't go out in that scene. (Andrew, North)

In towns where the number of local gay pubs and clubs was small, outreach work clearly impacted on social and sexual opportunities. In such towns, with few gay venues, it was often impossible to find places in which to socialise or have sex that were not also places of work:

> I think it's because this is such a small place anyway that it's inevitable that most of the people I see, if we do pub and club work, I'm going to have to drink with and socialise with. (Richard, Midlands)

> It's probably easier in a place like London where you've got access to so many venues, where you don't have to feel like after you've finished work you are still involved in it, because you're in the same place. Whereas here you cannot escape. It's a small scene. (Sean, North)

Although the size of the town made a difference, even workers in big cities could find it hard to maintain clear boundaries between work and their own personal life. This was because they were living and working in a community that was sexually defined (Edwards 1994). As Peter (East) said:

> [It's] more of an issue because it's not a geographical community, but a community gathered around sex … . The main link with people is sex. (Peter, East)

Several interviewees argued that because one of the main ways in which gay and bisexual workers expressed their links to the gay community was through having sex with other men, guidelines that restricted sexual behaviour carried a large personal cost:

> For a lot of gay men … their affiliation and participation in a gay community is about going out and cruising, and having sex, either in a PSE or a club, or a pub or whatever … . You participate in that community sexually as much as anything else … . A lot of gay men feel they've been recruited because they're gay … and then they sort of they feel like they're being told to stop being gay *(laughs)*. (Tim, London)

> When you do feel as if you want to go out and use a cruising area and you think 'No you can't' … you feel as if you've made this enormous sacrifice for the job. (Richard, Midlands)

Some interviewees therefore felt that their organisational codes of conduct invaded their private lives, and a few workers saw this as a form of repression:

> I mean there'll be a big fight in this office the day somebody tries to impose on us that we can't have a sex life [locally]. And I mean I would personally find that … completely unreasonable and quite frankly homophobic. (Edward, Midlands)

To understand why professional guidelines could raise such intense feelings, it is important to think more closely about the relationship between gay identity and sex. Some writers have highlighted the emphasis on sex amongst gay male communities (Stanley 1982), and for many gay men having sex both expresses their identity and links them to a community. The picture is of course complicated. Amongst outreach workers, it was clear that people felt differently about the relationship between having sex and their own sexual identity. For some, although sex was important, it did not necessarily form a major part of their sexual identity:

> I like having sex, I'm quite a sexual person, but having sex is not the most important part of my sexual identity, being free is. (Alex, London)

> I mean I think if I never have sex again I'll always be a gay man. (Toby, North)

Indeed for some people having sex was not a priority within their lives:

> Even though I've got a partner, I haven't [had] sex for at least two months … I

don't particularly like it. I don't think it's particularly important. (Craig, North)

You know, I wouldn't die tomorrow if I didn't have sex again. It's not a major part of my life at all; it's probably quite a minor part. If sex comes along fine. If I'm in the mood for it, I will you know, I'll accept it willingly. If I'm not I'll say no thank you. (Derek, London)

Even among those for whom having sex was felt to be personally important, many pointed out that this was not necessarily the case for all. For example, they knew other gay men who were celibate. In addition, the emphasis on sex within gay communities was seen as problematic by some. For example, Craig suggested that it was this that made him feel uncomfortable and out of place on the commercial gay scene:

My experience of gay male communities has been that they're very much geared towards sex and I think that's, for me, has done a lot of damage to those communities because … people are seen more as commodities than they are as individuals with feelings and with intelligence … . There's always these phases where you have these names for men … and they're quite degrading names. Like at one point it was 'piece of meat' or 'it', or you know 'that' … I just find it really, really horrible … . From how I see it, it's a large element of what gay communities are made up of. (Craig, North)

However, most male workers felt that having sex was extremely important to their own sense of sexual identity. This was particularly the case where their sexual identities were seen to be linked to the kinds of sex, or sexual partners, they had. For example:

K: And how important is having sex to your own sexual identity?

Oooohh! *(laughs)* God! *(smiles)* I think the honest answer for me is very, very, very, very, actually … I remember thinking yeah I'm gay, I'm gay now … when I had anal sex for the first time … . *(laughs)*. So I think it is actually. I mean I could theorise and come up with all sorts of conceptual bollocks and say not at all actually, my sexual identity is not about having sex. But actually it is, a lot. (Tim, London)

I feel more valid as a bisexual man if I'm having sex with a man and a woman … . If I didn't have sex with a man for five years, or I didn't have sex with a woman for five years, I would begin to lose a sense of my identity I think. (Nick, London)

Clearly, for many male workers having sex was linked to the ways in which they understood their self-identity, and could serve as a way to mark out their differences from others. Interestingly, sex was not spoken about this way by any of the women; however, this was not because they did not think sex was important:

> Oh it's [sex] very important! *(laughs)* … . Oh god yeah, I can't get enough of it! *(laughs)* I'm terrible. Poor [partner] he's exhausted! *(laughs)*. (Jill, South)

This general enjoyment of sex was very different to the ways in which many of the men frequently discussed having sex, in which a relationship between sex and a sense of community was made explicit:

> Well, we're in a sexualised culture and people, you know. The third question people ask is who you've slept with recently. You know, if you haven't got anyone to say you feel like a failure … . Sexual identity as a gay man is quite, you know … you *should* be doing it, and it's a bonding thing, and it's a key activity. And what type of sex you have, I mean that's very important being a gay man. (Jason, London)

For those men who strongly identified with the gay community or who saw having sex as central to their own sense of identity, or both, professional guidelines which restricted or limited the times, places and people with whom they could have sex had a major personal impact. For these men, work-related boundaries were frequently experienced as denying their sexuality; some found it hard to accept rules that they felt had a detrimental effect on their personal social and sexual lives.

Balancing organisational and personal needs

Most of the gay and bisexual workers stressed that they wanted the freedom to satisfy their own sexual needs, and a chance to socialise and explore their sexuality in a way that was unrelated to work. For this reason, it was important to 'have a sex life of their own'. However, many also felt a professional responsibility to protect the work they did and so had to balance their own needs with those of the organisation. This meant consciously managing their own social and sexual lives so as to carve out personal space:

> It's about me having a life, a social life and a sexual life, that is separate from work. Which I'm entitled to as anyone else to lead, no matter what that be. Whether it be illegal activities on a racecourse late at night *(smiles)*, or what have you. I'm as entitled to those choices as anyone else. So it's about making sure that I damn well get them, and that I don't feel restricted … I think for me [that's] the main reason for sort of trying to set my boundaries. (Rob, North)

One of the major problems faced by the workers was a lack of organisational support. Many spoke about their managers' anxiety over their social and sexual lives:

Boundary issues I suppose are the real problem with this sort of work. In the fact that you're working and socialising in the same area. I know our managers are very ... concerned ... scared that something could happen .... It's the inability to think of us as human beings that's the real problem – as sexual beings, especially through management structures. (Edward, Midlands)

However, despite such managerial concern, several workers felt their managers had not thought through the issues, and did not seem to understand the impact of such guidelines as 'no sex where you work'. It was suggested that the impact of living and working in the same community was not fully recognised. For example, the practical effects of guidelines, such as the expense incurred by having to travel to another town to drink or to meet sexual partners, were rarely considered. Workers found it particularly hard to talk about the dilemmas they faced if their managers did not understand the sexualised nature of the commercial gay scene, or workers' attachment to it. For this reason, interviewees were often critical of boundaries developed by those who were not gay men:

Are we working to the agenda of, quite often ... um ... workers who are not involved in the work, who do not fully understand the issues involved in cruising, and why people go cruising? .... And by workers who don't identify as gay or bisexual .... And from the female [manager's] side that's an even bigger issue. You know, whether they should be setting any agendas for gay men's work? I don't believe they should. (Derek, London)

What makes it difficult? [to draw boundaries] I think primarily it's like fear. You know, the management don't understand, especially if they're not gay, or have no idea what it's like to be, to be gay. And sort of, you know, sexually active in that sort of sense .... Some people in the health service like to turn around and say 'Well you do not sleep with people who perceive you to be a health worker'. Fine, for them that viewpoint might be great, they don't sleep with patients. Fine. But it's not really acceptable to me .... That boundary is so ridiculous that it's impossible to work within that framework. (Richard, Midlands)

A few gay male workers felt, probably erroneously, that if they were heterosexual they would not be asked to keep sexual boundaries. They were angry that boundaries were pushed on them with no recognition of the different effects they may have because of their sexuality, the nature of the gay scene and the relationship of both to the nature of their work.

Who can be a sexual partner?

The guidelines that projects had developed around the work often directly affected whom the workers were able to have sex with. For example, it was common that workers would not be allowed to use the places where they worked to meet sexual partners. This could be frustrating:

> A lot of places I socialise in are [local] so does that mean anybody I've seen who recognises me from the cruising site I cannot go with? ... I don't know how many people we've seen this year on Cruise Project, but last year we saw well over 2000 people. Does that mean all those 2000 people if they all recognise me I would not be able to have any sort of personal interaction with them? Then if that's the case it's wrong, the system's got to be wrong. (Derek, London)

> I was single and I did want to find a partner and stuff like that and ... my client group were potentially people who could be, people who I could either have sex with, or perhaps become partners or whatever. And that was an issue for me because you know it was affecting the way I felt about myself ... I felt like my work was coming before my own personal [life] ... . So, it was a dilemma and the alternative was to go out of town. But then that became a problem as well, in terms of financing it and also the time it took, and the effort just to go out. (Isaac, Midlands)

As the major organisational guideline in relation to sexual boundaries was not to have sex with 'clients', a significant issue was the definition of who exactly was a client. This was discussed a great deal, and for some workers this distinction was far from clear:

> What is a client and what isn't? I mean if it's everybody that you've ever had any contact with ... whether they've spoken to you or not, then that makes it very difficult to assess who hasn't, especially because everybody's had access to the condom racks (in pubs) and things like that. (Sean, North)

The variation in the kinds of men met through outreach work meant that for workers a large part of developing boundaries involved deciding who exactly counted as a client (this process is discussed in the next chapter). For this reason, outreach work clearly affected where and with whom workers had sex. The fact that some workers had interpreted their guidelines to mean that they could only have sex with people from outside the area where they worked meant that they now had to travel for sex. This was mentioned by some interviewees as the biggest effect of the work.

When interviewees did socialise or have sex and work in the same place, some felt that this communicated confusing signals to others. As George explained:

> How do you communicate those boundaries to people who the night before, you know, you said: 'Oh we can't possibly be sort of having sex', whatever. And then the night afterwards, they see you cruising somebody, or picking up someone in a club, or whatever. And how you can legitimise that? (George, North)

Although a few workers felt that men they came into contact with through out-reach work found it easy to understand their role, others raised issues such as not being seen to favour some men, or damaging men's self esteem by turning down their offers of sex and then being seen to have sex with someone else. As service providers, they were keen to emphasise issues of equity and responsibility. Workers were also concerned not to damage their credibility by being seen to have sex with clients:

> I remember an instance where somebody who is a member of the social group, who I supplied them with condoms, took it upon himself to invite himself round to my house ... and we ended up in bed. And then after that, I was like agonised ... about, you know. 'God, this guy could be perceived as a client'. And then somebody who runs that social group sort of turned around at a party a few weeks later and said, you know: 'Are you still running around screwing everybody?' And I thought ... I must be seen as a real sort of monster or what-ever. You know, I seduced this guy ... . But you know from my point of view, this guy had actually actively sought me out ... . You know *he'd* driven across the city you know and been quite persistent. (Richard, Midlands)

Richard further feared that if he explained what had actually happened he could be breaking boundaries in terms of confidentiality.

Apart from not having sex with existing service users, for some men a further issue arose, namely that of having sex with *potential* future clients. Being part of the local gay community meant that this could easily occur. Workers often felt very vulnerable and were anxious that any mistake they made could reflect badly on their work. There was a fear of exposing themselves to charges of professional misconduct if they had sex with local gay or bisexual men. Therefore, their work and personal lives bore a complicated relationship to one another. As Edward put it, 'Your social life is the bit that keeps you sane. And yet it potentially is the bit that really screws you up'. For those working in small towns this dilemma was especially acute, and interviewees were often concerned that they did not stop men accessing the services that they needed:

> If I go out and, you know, just sort of pick somebody up and things. You're still partly the professional ... even though they haven't been a client at that point. You think: 'Well would they use the service at a later date 'cos they've slept with the worker?' (Richard, Midlands)

Meeting sexual contacts in settings that were also their places of work could make workers anxious about their professional reputation. Where they were the only worker in a town this situation was made more complicated. Here, if the out-reach worker became sexually involved with a service user there may be no other colleague to refer them to.

Working when socialising

Working and socialising or having sex in the same places meant that people often reported feeling they were always at work. They described how it was often hard to relax on the gay scene because they would be constantly thinking about work. For example, when out for an evening with friends, they might start having ideas for future campaigns, or find themselves checking to see if there were condoms in pubs or clubs. Places of leisure thus became places of work:

> It also means that when it comes to your own social life, and you have a night off, that you don't feel like going out. You don't feel like having a social life, you don't feel as though you can unwind. Because it's ... the connotation is where you are going is work. So there are those problems. (Edward, Midlands)

Furthermore, because of being known, and conscious of the need to remain credible, workers felt they had to be continually on guard when socialising in workplaces. For example:

> I was at the [pub] a few weeks ago and they had a stripper on, and this guy was wandering through the crowd and he's like molesting the guy next to me. I thought 'Oh that's fine'. And then he got hold of me and I'm thinking, you know, 'I hope he doesn't go too far 'cos I'm surrounded by about 500 of my client group. You know, if he like pulls me trousers down or something how can I have the respect of these people?' ... I have absolutely no wish to have my trousers ripped off in front of 500 people that I've got to work with and relate to on a professional basis ... . But you know that's the sort of position you're in. You know you're going out socially but you're always conscious of what *might* happen. And you're developing strategies in your mind all the time about how you'd deal with it if it ever did. (Roger, Midlands)

> I'm conscious that my actions are limited in some ways. I mean, if I go and act like a complete prat at a club it's going to be difficult to go back and enter that environment again as a professional ... . For that reason you never stop working. (Andrew, North)

Female interviewees felt that retaining a professional identity when socialising with gay men was easier because there was less potential for role confusion. Their boundaries were also less likely to be challenged by service users:

> I do not want sex with, with gay men right? So when I go out socially, and they come and talk to me ... and ... [ask a question] I can say: 'Yes it is', or 'I'm not sure, I'll find out, when are you next here?' And they go, because there's none of this play between us, the sexual play with the conversation. Whereas with the boys, that question could be seen as being tantamount to a chat up

line, or a way of getting into their company. So that makes it quite difficult for them. Whereas for me it's not. They can stay and talk to me all evening if they want to but I'm not going to end up having sex with them. (Sandi, East)

Workers felt boundary making was necessary because of some service users' reluctance to distinguish between the times when they were socialising and working. A common complaint in the interviews was being approached and asked to discuss gay, HIV, or safer sex issues when socialising. One worker described this situation as like being part of the royal family: 'You lose your privacy'. Most encountered a tension between keeping their social lives private and maintaining an image of being accessible and friendly. For this reason, many said that they did not feel able to ignore (potential) service users when socialising:

[I] make up my mind and say: 'Well I'm not working, and if anyone comes up to me … then I'll tell them I'm not working'. And you sit there and you think: 'OK that's going to be really easy to do'. It's not … . And if the conversation you're involved in with a group of friends is like, about something that is relevant to your work, and someone thinks you're there to work, and so they come along and they join in. And [then] they start asking all sorts of questions. It's like very difficult to explain … . 'I'm not actually working, fuck off', you know *(laughs)*. (Rob, North)

Most workers emphasised that because of the overlap between work and leisure, they could not always be as frank or rude in dealing with unwarranted interruptions as they would have liked. Even in their leisure time, workers were thus continually aware of their role, and felt that they had a duty to represent their organisation. This meant having to be polite all the time:

The most explicit example of that is the club owners cornering me when I'm not working, which I would say happens 50 per cent of the times I'm in there … . And there even more there's pressure to listen. And I can't just say: 'I'm not working tonight' to them because there's always pressure … to make sure we have access to the men inside their club. And that's really made like, quite spoiled my evening a couple of times. (Toby, North)

If I was just a gay man in [the town] and there was somebody I didn't like I would feel quite happy about telling them I didn't like them. And I would make it very obvious, and very clear. As workers we're prevented from doing that. You can't be seen to alienate individuals, I mean it's obviously not on. And we quite often find ourselves having our ears bent by people who are, you know doing our heads in for hours on end in a club … . I personally find it a real strain having to talk to people I don't like. Especially when it's in your time and not work time. So, you know that's a pain. (Edward, Midlands)

Maintaining good relationships, whether working or not, was felt to be vital to the success of outreach work. As 'professionals', workers were never off duty.

One of the concerns expressed about drawing very rigid boundaries between work and leisure was that sometimes useful work-related information would be discovered when out socialising. Choosing to socialise elsewhere meant that workers could miss out on important conversations. As Rob said:

> If I avoid the pub altogether, apart from [when I'm] working, then I miss out a lot on what's happening ... . Someone came up to me the other week in the pub: 'Do you know that there's a chap down the river bank who's taking chaps home and robbing them when they're cruising? He's a young chap.' [He] gave me a description [and] I said: 'I know him, yes I do. I've met him.' And that information was of course very useful for working with men I know cottage or cruise ... . But if I set very rigid stuff [boundaries] I [would] miss out on all that ... I think it's better to be part of the community than [to be] out of it. (Rob, North)

Workers reported becoming increasingly annoyed with people approaching them when socialising, and described the need to limit interactions so that they did not feel trapped by their work:

> To start with you go in with this huge amount of energy and you think you know like: 'Yeah, it's gonna be brill'. Then you really start to get very pissed off with people who will ... when you're sat in a pub with some friends ... who will engage you in a conversation ... . It's only sort of as it develops and the initial energy perhaps has gone, or you're trying to be stricter about things for your own protection, that you really start getting angry and annoyed, and frustrated with what's happening. (Rob, North)

> On a personal level, the boundaries are there so I'm not swamped really ... . The thing I'm really quite good at now, which I wasn't at the beginning, is actually when people come and talk to me in a pub when I'm not working, to say: 'I'm not working, you can see me on Monday'. And [I'm] not feeling guilty about that any more.

> *K:*   How have you managed to change, to do that?

> Well it just got to a ridiculous situation really! Where people were spoiling my evenings ... . You know, I was out with friends and then these other people came up and [tried to] hijack my time. (George, North)

The passage of time affected workers' appreciation of the need for boundaries. Many learned the importance of having interests separate from work, and time to themselves. Some felt that establishing boundaries became easier with time as their projects became known and there was less pressure to involve people in the work.

Immersed in the work

One of the reasons why work was felt to impact so much on social life was personal involvement in it. Many workers were guided by a desire to help their peers and so reported finding it hard to say no to people who needed information:

> Quite often problems are presented as urgencies, or people are desperate, or they're just really depressed ... . Obviously, it's difficult to turn that sort of person away ... . Like I say, it's not a job it's a way of life really in the end. (Edward, Midlands)

As members of a shared community, workers often found it hard not to provide information to people even though they were not working. In this way, their experiences were not unlike others doing community based work (Cruikshank 1989). Part of the problem was that the workers felt responsible to pass on information that could save people's lives:

> It's the emotive part isn't it? That's what makes it difficult. The fact that if you don't answer that question that person may do something that's unsafe that night. And that could be the, the one instance and he's HIV positive or whatever else ... . That's the biggest one [fear] for everyone. (Sandi, East)

The feeling that they had to be constantly available to provide support made it hard for some workers to maintain a separate personal life. Some reported having to cancel leisure plans to deal with a crisis:

> On one occasion, [my co-worker] and I were working, and we were in a club and there was a very distressed client. And like, the bar staff were sort of begging and pleading for us to help this guy ... . And we had to get this guy admitted to psychiatric hospital for his own safety. Because he was sort of threatening to kill himself and he was very, very distressed. And we were like sort of ostensibly on duty from half seven to eleven. But at like two o'clock in the morning we're still sitting in this psychiatric hospital trying to persuade them to admit him ... . So there's sort of no predictability about it. It's very difficult to make arrangements socially to do anything. (Roger, Midlands)

Others found it very difficult to switch off from work and the issues involved. This meant that it was often hard to wind down (Hochschild 1983). Part of the reason here was the work itself had become 'a way of life'. For example, issues of sexuality, safer sex and HIV permeated respondents' leisure time:

> Some of the situations that I'm involved in are so emotive and stuff. I don't know, I just find it really, really difficult to switch off. And I think a lot of people in this profession suffer from exactly the same thing. I think the only

real interest in our lives, apart from going on the scene ... is work. And everything's based around work, or is connected with work. (Toby, North)

This experience of being caught up in work has been highlighted in other studies
of community based workers (Cruikshank 1989). But for gay and bisexual workers, the tensions appeared to be heightened because they were working with other
men who have sex with men. This meant that many of the issues they were dealing
with in work also touched them personally. Indeed a few suggested that they sometimes over-empathised with the community, which caused their personal lives to
suffer. As Sean put it:

> You become kind of obsessed with the work. I mean there are some times
> when I just don't, I never want to see another gay man. Do you know what I
> mean? Like for a week or so. Just because you've mixed with so many and
> you've talked about all the same things all over and over again ... . Enough is
> enough ... . You take on all of the negativity around like safer sex, and peo-
> ple's attitudes to gay men, and you take it back [home] with you. And [then]
> your partners get it and suffer. (Sean, North)

Sean went on to say that in order to stay sane he needed to find time when he did
not think about sex and sexuality. As well as feeling fed-up of talking about 'gay
issues', a minority of the men interviewed said they had started to have negative
feelings about gay men. As George explained:

> In this job you do see the worst bits of the community really. Sometimes I just
> go home and think: 'God I hate it, I hate it ... gay men are just disgustingly
> horrible'. You know they're abusive, and all the rest of it. (George, North)

At least two men described these feelings, somewhat jokingly, as 'becoming
homophobic'. One talked about how he and his co-worker would find themselves
making comments about 'prissy queens' simply as a way of dealing with these
feelings. Another man said these feelings had led him to not find gay men sexually
attractive any more. Elsewhere, Cruikshank (1989) has suggested that feelings of
hostility towards users are classic signs of burnout among community based workers and signal a need for time off. However, negative feelings about sex were also
related to the fact that for many men sex was now associated with work.

Lusty yet bored

Working in sexually charged environments; talking about sex all day; or thinking
about it but not being allowed to have it; made some workers very frustrated. As
Keith put it: 'It would be nice to take my work [home] with me in that sense'. This
phenomenon even led workers to say they felt jealous of people who were having
sex:

I feel resentful that people talk about having lots of sex when I'm not. [I] feel I'm Mr Safe Sex and boring. They are having fun. (Peter, East)

'Working with sex all day' was felt by some to have had a negative impact on their personal lives. For example, one gay man said that he no longer wanted to talk at home about sex or his own sexual experiences. Others felt that work had 'taken the magic out of sex' for them:

> It is an intensive sexual environment that I work in, and that also has the effect of in some ways demystifying sex, and what sex is, and making it less exciting and less interesting and more, more to do with my work. (Nick, London)

For many people, sex is seen as something different from work, a marker for leisure. However, for those involved in sex work, or work with sex, this is often not the case. Angie Hart (1992) mentions this in her ethnography of prostitutes' clients in Spain. She describes how for prostitutes 'trips out' were seen as an escape from the daily routine. As such, the women (her emphasis):

> did not like to talk about their work. When one prostitute, Antonia, began to discuss men's penises – *a work related topic* – during a coach trip to Lourdes, she was quickly silenced by other prostitutes who were on the trip.
>
> (Hart 1992:204)

Similarly, for many outreach workers sex was no longer an experience so very different to work. Indeed, some described how sex had become work and, as such, the meanings attached to it had changed. For these men sex did not serve to relieve stress and revive spirits (Lippert 1977; Nickolay 1991). After talking about sex all day it could be the last thing workers wanted, a situation which often infuriated their partners. A further reported reason for the work having a negative effect on workers' sex lives was derived from continually seeing or hearing about the negative side of sex. As Nick mentioned:

> You're dealing with people's problems around identity, and their traumas and stresses and that takes its toll actually … . That's made me very aware of the pitfalls of sex and sexuality, and sexual identity. And the shit that people have in their minds around it. And I find that very depressing. (Nick, London)

How outreach work impacted on people's sex lives was obviously related to their own sexuality and the sex they had. For example, Jill, a straight woman, described how working with female sex workers had been more destructive to her own sexual relationship than working with gay men. It had caused her to question aspects of male heterosexuality and raised questions about her partner's potential use of sex workers.

A space of one's own

As mentioned above, boundaries were felt by interviewees to be important by providing a chance to 'switch off', and in ensuring there was life outside work. Some workers even suggested that unless they took time out for themselves they would 'go off their trolley, completely':

> Basically my home at the end of the day is an escape … I'm allowed to just be a couch potato … . When I'm just vegetating on go the jogging bottoms, I can sort of crack the gel out of my hair and just be me. (Steve, North)

It was interesting that workers talked about needing 'space to be me' or feeling that they had to make a choice between 'me and work'. In this way, boundaries offered a different kind of protection to that discussed in the previous chapter where the emphasis was on protecting the work. Here boundaries were talked about in terms of their importance for mental health:

> I mean sometimes you hear of gay men's workers up and down the country, you know, like they complain about their boundaries, that they can't do this and they can't do that, and they haven't got the sexual autonomy to do what they like, and all the rest of it. And in reality they [the boundaries] are there to stop that outreach worker going loopy … . The fact that we do so much intensive work throughout a week has actually brought it home to us a lot quicker than it has with people who maybe only go out [outreaching] once a week … . They never have that much exposure to clients and therefore … boundary issues are just this millstone round their neck to them, that are preventing them from doing this that and the other. In reality we've reached a stage where the boundary issues are actually keeping us sane. (Edward, Midlands)

Some interviewees mentioned that that they would become boring if all they did was work, and others feared burnout. This meant that the importance of doing something different to work was frequently stressed. As Keith said:

> I mean something that I have tried to introduce is like things for me that's totally sort of like got nothing to do with work, got nothing to do with my sexuality … . That would be something maybe that I would recommend to anybody. You know as a complete break from everything. You know, making rugs! … things that take your mind off completely. (Keith, North)

And as Nick commented:

> It's important to see where your work starts and finishes, and it's important to have … a life apart from your work, and that's a personal boundary. But it's also a boundary we expect of people to display when we interview people. And that's about avoiding burnout. (Nick, London)

Interestingly, those workers who had lots of heterosexual friends, or did not socialise a lot on the commercial gay scene (or both), reported finding it easier to draw boundaries. Having a social life outside the gay community was important in enabling them to differentiate between their work and personal lives. For those whose personal and work lives revolved around the same places and activities, establishing clear boundaries was obviously much more difficult.

'What do you have to do to get a shag in this town?': occupation and sexual partners

The nature of their occupation had very specific effects on men's sex lives. Numerous examples were recounted about how, because of their job, they were seen variously as 'frigid'; 'safer sex gurus'; 'safer sex police', or even HIV positive by other gay community members. This affected their ability to obtain sexual partners. Some male gay and bisexual workers reported that one of the positive effects of being an HIV worker was that they were seen to be glamorous, knowledgeable and safe. This sometimes made them more attractive to other men:

> It's partly because we portray ourselves as sexy to make men want to get involved with us, or take what we have to offer. And it's partly about [them] ... seeing us as people who are confident about sex, who know about sex, who emotionally and physically are safe to have sex with ... I think in a community where a lot of people are perhaps coming to terms with what kind of sex, sex is for them ... and perhaps insecure about homosexual sex ... there's this notion that we're confident, sorted, able to do it nice and easily, and I suppose look after people almost at some level. And so that makes them feel emotionally safe. That we're not going to abuse that relationship, and that they're going to have a satisfying experience. (Nick, London)

> I think the minute you're an HIV worker people want to have sex with you .... Because you're just having the kinds of conversations about sex that people never get to have .... They want to get their hands on some of that candour, and some of that apparent calmness, and frankness, and worked-out-ness about sex .... People really want that. (Tim, London)

Certainly, their occupation made many workers well known and, for some, this expanded their sexual network. Having more sexual partners was partly a result of meeting more people. However, the economic aspects of paid work meant that some could also afford to socialise more, or to go abroad where they felt freer to have more sex than they did locally. To some degree these experiences may be related to the fact that many of the men were in their early twenties and enjoying the opportunities brought by being young and single. However, the nature of their work was obviously also relevant.

For some interviewees the impact of work was different and sex itself became more important. They spoke about having 'lots of sex as a way to forget about work' (Toby), or mentioned the importance of having good sex to counteract the negative stories they often heard whilst working. Indeed, some interviewees felt that having a good sexual relationship gave them personal support. Having a person-centred job supporting others increased the need to have someone to listen, and to remind them that sex and relationships could be good. In this regard, those with pre-existing sexual relationships often found it easier to draw boundaries between work and other parts of their lives because they had a more clearly defined personal life and demands on their time outside of work.

The effects on people's sex lives were variable. In addition to the positive changes brought by their occupation, the nature of the work could also make it harder to meet sexual partners. A few male gay and bisexual workers said that people were scared of having sex with them because of 'what we might uncover in their sexuality'; or because they did not know how to put a condom on; or thought the worker must be HIV positive:

> It's like, they're putting a condom on and they were going: 'God, I was convinced you were going to look at me when I was doing that!' You know. And I'm going, well, you know: 'No I wasn't looking and I'm not interested' ... I mean that really brings it home to you. You've got to the stage where, you're in a very intimate situation with one person and they're like having kittens because you might be looking at how they're putting a condom on ... . If you've got to that stage you'd think that they'd have put your occupation to one side, but its not always the case. (Edward, Midlands)

> If you work for an HIV agency people always think you have HIV ... and it does fucking ruin your sex life, because they won't approach you because they think you're HIV positive. (Sanjay, Midlands)

A few workers talked specifically about approaching strangers when looking for sexual partners as: 'It's easier to start from scratch with them, rather than having preconceived ideas about who you are, and what you are, because they know what you do for a living.' As George explained:

> I very rarely sleep with men in this city and that is for all sorts of reasons .... A lot of it is about fear that they want to have sex with me because of my job. You know 'Mr Safer Sex' and all that stuff. And the other fear is that they may tell other people in the city what I'm like in bed really. And this is this person who keeps saying how wonderful safer sex is and how erotic it is, and they may not find me very erotic at all, find me quite a bore! That feels, you know, that feels quite difficult. (George, North)

A few men reported that their occupation had made their experience of sex much more clinical. For example, George felt that the psychological barriers he put up when talking about sex at work were hard to break down on a personal level (see also Hochschild 1983). He had trained himself not to have sexual feelings when working and felt this had started to continue into his own sex life:

> I'm a lot more aware of the way I have sex. I'm not talking about like safer sex or anything, but it's actually just sex really. And it, it feels a lot less spontaneous than it was. It's almost as though I've become a technician really. And again that pressure on being this sort of incredible erotic, safer sex person who can spread cream over people, you know. OK, that's all a bit of fun but I've got sheets, I'm not going to spread cream all over you! So that feels very difficult, that's a very, very personal level. I think it has changed the way I have sex. (George, North)

Thus, although George now felt more in control sexually, he felt he had lost any sexual spontaneity.

Work affected sexual relationships in other ways. For example, by having to deal with partners' jealousy when working in sexual spaces, or by playing a supportive or counselling role in relation to partners' anxieties. One man said that intense conversations about his work had led his lover to question his own sexuality and what he wanted from the relationship. More commonly, workers found themselves dealing with their partner's HIV-related concerns. Some felt frustrated that as a result their own sex lives seemed to be turning into work:

> That has happened you know, that's actually led to some pretty intensive disclosures about themselves. About, you know, maybe a time when they were very drunk, or very in lust, and maybe did something that was totally unsafe … I suppose to a point I can put it on one side … I have actually been in that situation where I have like put it on one side, and I'm sort of like trying to carry on and sort of re-arouse them. And they're like 'No, No' and getting really upset about it. And it's so frustrating. And I'm not always as sensitive as I'd like to be because … it is sometimes important for me to think with my dick rather than my head yeah? … I just want to have like a good time and that's not possible. (Keith, North)

When discussing sex-related issues, it was hard for some men to keep work out of their conversations, for example, by making reference to sexual surveys and research when discussing issues in their personal relationships. Workers could also find themselves being accused of professionalising their own relationships. I have encountered such experiences myself, with partners 'not wanting to have a theoretical discussion' about sex-related issues. Living in a culture where sex is often portrayed as liberating, instinctual and uncontrollable (see also Schover 1989) it is perhaps not surprising that having a very rational, calm, work-related focus can make sex, and related discussions, seem very different.[1]

Safer sexual practices

Working in HIV prevention led many workers to reflect on their own sexual practices. For some, the work directly led to their having more safer sex, although this was not the case for all. Others felt the work had made them over-aware of HIV-related risks which could cause panic or put them off sex:

> [Work] has had a huge effect on the type of sex that I would have, and stuff like that. Basically because I'm in a position where I get … regular information about people with HIV, people with AIDS and stuff like that. So yeah, that has a big effect and it frightens me … . And because I'm constantly thinking about it, it's not something I can put in the back of my mind … I'm less interested in sex because of that. (Craig, North)

Anxieties about sex were particularly likely where workers felt responsible for safer sex. In instances such as these, they spoke about feeling they were always at work and unable to shake off their safer sex role. For some, the pressure on their sex lives and activities was further complicated by feeling that their professional credibility would be damaged if they were known to practice unsafe sex:

> That is a pressure … somebody saying: 'Oh I had it with that [worker] we had unsafe sex'. And what would that do to your reputation? (Sanjay, Midlands)

Where there was a small and closely networked gay scene interviewees felt that their own sexual experiences had the potential to damage their professional identity. This was an area where they felt it was impossible to draw a personal and professional boundary: if it became known that they had unsafe sex, their professionalism would be seriously challenged. In this regard, it is interesting to note that the job advertisement for two of the men I interviewed specified that all applicants had to be personally committed to practising safer sex.

Others felt that the idea that they should always have safer sex was wrong. For example, it was suggested that the important issue was whether or not they had used their power as a worker in order to have unsafe sex. A few men also felt that it was important to recognise that they were as likely to 'make mistakes' as other gay men. More generally, there has been a recognition amongst some gay men's workers of the need for more open discussion about the times when they have had unsafe sex, rather than feeling ashamed about it (Gorna 1996; Whinnery 1993). However, for many men interviewed, admitting to unsafe sex when they spend their working lives telling others about its dangers proved extremely difficult.

More confident and understanding

A very common theme amongst the gay male outreach workers was that the work had made them feel more confident in their sexual encounters. This meant that they felt more able to say what they wanted and liked in sexual relationships, including saying no:

> I've become so much more assertive around sex and the sex I want ... I remember one particular man I sort of got home, and basically all he wanted to do was have anal sex, you know without asking or anything really .... And it's the first time that I've actually told somebody to get out of the bed and get dressed and go, you know. And before I'd never have done that. I would have tried to placate him, and said: 'Oh no, we can do lots of other things instead'. But it was 'No'. If that's all he's into what's the point really. And he went! (George, North)

This new assertiveness was felt to be a direct result of having acquired the skills needed in outreach work. For example, as Jason and Andrew explained:

> I'm also more assertive now, and I can say I don't find it [anal sex] comfortable. And they say: 'Yeah but if you use poppers etc.' And I say 'Well I'd just rather not.' Partly because I've grown up, but partly because I've been involved in a field where we're dealing with sex, and I've learnt to just be more assertive. (Jason, London)

> You're always saying to people you know: 'Talk about sex, say what you want', and I can do that now. Whereas before I'd feel embarrassed ... I've become a lot more sort of playful and don't take it [sex] so seriously .... And I think that's a result of talking about it a lot. (Andrew, North)

Greater confidence came from practising skills used in work such as talking about sex, negotiating safer sex and relationships, and discussing different personal experiences. Of course, some of this developing confidence could be related to increasing sexual experience and maturity. However, comments about confidence were not restricted to the younger workers.

A further way in which work impacted on people's personal lives was through making them more knowledgeable about safer sex, public sex environments, sexuality, sexual techniques and the medical aspects of HIV. This probably has parallels with most occupations. Over time, work-related knowledge is built up and new awareness and expertise developed. This increased sensitivity made some feel 'more liberated and worldly'. Their greater understanding of a wide variety of sexual practices, for example, meant that different sexual activities had become normalised for them. Having more experience and understanding also made some men more tolerant:

> I've seen such a spectrum of what people's sexualities are, from people who are celibate, to people who, I don't know, do what might be considered the most bizarre and perverse things. And they've all been normalised for me in a way, because they're familiar .... It's removed a lot of assumptions for me as

well: who has sex; what kinds of sex; and what their identity is ... I don't feel the need for somebody who has sex, homosexual sex to identify as gay or bisexual, whereas I would've done before ... . But yeah it's normalised a huge spectrum of sexual activity. And I think that's been very positive. (Nick, London)

Generally speaking, people spoke about 'having their eyes opened through outreach work which led to a greater tolerance and understanding. They had come to appreciate the differences between men, rather than seeing them as a homogenous group. Some also felt more relaxed and open to trying out different kinds of sexual activities themselves. This was in part because they had been made more aware of other sexual and relationship possibilities. For a few, knowledge of different sexual tastes made it easier to talk about sex outside work and, in some cases, to be more helpful or tolerant of others.

More valid sexuality

Undertaking HIV prevention outreach had different effects on people's sexualities. On a positive note, many of the men interviewed stated that the work had empowered them:

On the sexuality side, yes this work's actually done wonders for me ... . You know working at a project that solely worked with male sex workers, where talking about sex was breakfast lunch and tea. And literally it *was* while you was eating, you know. Then I have no difficulty talking about sex ... . And what I think really has highlighted it for me was working at [SaferCruising] and meeting young 16 and 17 years olds who although they'd yeah, they'd got a lot of other issues, were quite clear about their sexuality. They was able to talk about sex in a mature and adult way, and talk about sexual practices ... . That's done me the world of good. And whatever happens in the future I'm glad I came into this work just for that. (Derek, London)

For this man, being able to talk about sex and sexuality without being embarrassed had led to his coming out as bisexual. In this way, he felt that his own sexuality had been validated through his work experiences. On a different note, one of the Asian workers said his confidence in his sexuality meant that he had decided he would never get married, despite cultural pressures to do so. For others, doing the work had encouraged them to be more open about sexual activities that they had kept secret before. One man reported having developed 'Cottage Queen Pride' as a result of his work, and talked about how he had become more open about his own use of PSEs as he no longer felt that it was something to feel guilty or ashamed of. Many gay and bisexual men described how being employed because of their sexuality was enormously validating. For those who had had many negative experiences in the past, this was obviously hugely important, and many felt that they had blossomed as a result.

Significantly, for one of the straight women and a bisexual male worker in a relationship with a woman this was not the case. Nick felt that working in a gay and bisexual outreach project had validated his sex with men but not with women. He felt that becoming involved in this work had made him 'hugely aware of his sexuality' because it made it more visible to others. The positive side of this was that his bisexual identity was made obvious to people who only knew he had a female partner. However, the down side was that he found it difficult to have his relationship with his female partner acknowledged at work:

> I'm now very politicised, I'm very queer identified and very networked in that community, and very politicised around my identity. And I'm very, very aware of that. And I'm also in a very male environment, and a very male sexual environment and that is quite threatening I think … . And that's put a strain on our relationship … . It took a year and a half before somebody [at work] said they'd like to meet her for instance … . You know, this is the most important person in my life and it's taken them a year and a half to respect that they even exist. (Nick, London)

The fact that sex with women is somewhat of a taboo topic amongst gay men did not help this situation.

Friendships

A frequent example given of the breakdown in the boundary between work and personal life was when talking to friends. Many interviewees said they found it hard not to discuss work-related issues in social conversations. For some, this link between their personal and work life was often exaggerated because of the overlap between the local gay and HIV prevention communities. Many interviewees described socialising with colleagues, and several workers knew very personal information about others in the HIV prevention field. For example, as Jason described when finding out who was going to be his new manager:

> He's coming to this job which is quite high position on the management team and I have copies of [safer sex cards showing] his penis. And I know he has sex in seedy clubs. And I know he gets off his head on Ecstasy. (Jason, London)

The integration of gay and HIV prevention networks meant that personal and professional lives were often linked through gossip and friendships. Interviewees often had to work with friends or past sexual contacts and many made reference to the networked and 'incestuous' nature of HIV prevention work. This meant that work and personal lives often took on 'a very mixed feel'. Boundaries were important to help workers judge what to say about work, and to not reveal personal information to their friends about people they had met.

For some workers, talking about sex became 'matter of fact' and they expressed anxiety that by discussing their work, or talking about sex in great detail when

Advantages (boundary)	Disadvantages (barrier)
Imposes or gives air of professionalism	Always seen as a professional
Gives work structure	Can unnecessarily restrict work
Defines roles and relationships	Roles too inflexible
Preserves confidentiality	Obstructs sharing of information
Stops abuse of service users	Limits relationships because of professional role
Encourages trust between service user and worker	Creates a false sense of security
Helps set goals	Goals framed by workers' needs
Provides legal protection	Limits effectiveness (e.g. by having to work with the legal age of consent)
Provides a safe space for others to talk	
Identifies personal space for workers	Restricts use of social venues
Gives workers confidence and support	Discourages creativity
Ensures equal opportunities	Creates distance from service users
Empowers service users	
Stops unwanted intrusion	Creates social barriers
Helps avoid burnout	
Builds trust	
Helps prevent damaging gossip	
Helps provide a good service through a focus on work	Psychological barriers hard to break down in your own time

Figure 2 Advantages and disadvantages of having boundaries.

socialising they were seen to be behaving outrageously. Many felt they had become blasé about sex (see also Grey 1993) and so were more 'up-front and crude' about it within their friendships. They no longer got embarrassed but tended to talk about sex in a clinical and detached fashion. In fact, many felt that they now thought about sex in a different way to other people, and that this affected the kinds of conversations they had with friends. Some workers felt that these changes meant that they had begun to talk to their friends as professionals rather than peers:

I think once you go into this work ... that's something you have to accept, that you're gonna be seen as being the expert .... Once you start this work, who's a client and who's a friend? 'Cos you talk to anybody about safer sex, anybody you can because that's your job. (Sandi, East)

On the other hand, when workers talked to friends about sex as a peer they could feel that they had not provided a good service. For example, Isaac reported feeling very guilty after telling a friend 'not to be ridiculous' when he expressed anxiety about a sexual encounter, and talked about going for an HIV test. Although he felt his friend was not at risk, he was concerned that he would have reacted in a more supportive manner if this anxiety had been addressed to him in a work context.

A final way in which work affected friendships arose from the barriers that had to be created in work contexts. Some interviewees found it hard keeping friends at a distance when working, particularly when they met them in a club, pub or PSE:

People say, oh you know: 'You're talking to us, [but] your eyes are wandering as well, 'cos you're not [really] interested' ... . How can I explain to them working in here [sauna], I have to keep my eyes and ears open all the time. It's very hard. (Sanjay, Midlands)

The other problem with like boundaries is the people who do know you socially, when you are working will come up and have a drink with you. So you could be like trying to give out, whatever you're giving out, and you know you've got this, this mate at the side of you who's like sort of trying to tell you about what they've been doing that week. It's a real pain. (Richard, Midlands)

Living and working in the same community made such crossovers inevitable and many men found it hard to distance themselves from people they knew socially.

Conclusions

You've got basically your social life and your work life, and in the end both affect each other. And whether that should happen, I mean obviously in theory, in terms of a job it should never happen, but in reality in this job, I mean it's impossible to not make it happen. (Edward, Midlands)

This chapter has explored some of the links between sex, sexuality and work to explain why boundaries were felt to be important. Far from being clearly separate, workers experienced the different aspects of their lives as being joined in complex ways. In this way, their experiences contradict the work of those such as Seidler (1991) who has argued that modern life involves a forced separation of identities between home and work:

It is very possible in an urban world not to mix socially with people at work. So it becomes possible to maintain 'different identities' in the different parts of our lives.

(Seidler 1991:115).

Having said this, workers did feel that having boundaries was important, even if their enthusiasm for them was tempered by an awareness of the issues they created. In the interviews and workshop conducted as part of this study, a range of positive reasons for having boundaries was identified. These included: protecting the project or work, preventing unwanted intrusion by workers to clients and *vice versa*, avoiding burnout and building trust. But boundaries were also seen as leading to difficulties upon occasion. They might, for example, distance workers from the local gay community, create a false sense of security and restrict work practices. Figure 2 on page 98 offers a summary of the perceived advantages and disadvantages. Overall, for the individuals in this study boundary creation and maintenance was seen as an essential yet problematic process.

Part 3

How boundaries are made

Having explored the reasons why boundaries are seen to be important but not always easy to maintain, this part of the book describes in detail the ways in which they are made. Chapter 6 discusses the processes by which workers interviewed learned to make boundaries, and describes the different methods that they used. Chapter 7 shows how ideas about being professional guided workers' boundary making within work, and between work and other parts of their lives.

6 Boundary work

Unlike in more established professions, there was rarely a pre-existing set of guidelines which HIV prevention outreach workers agreed to abide by as a condition of their employment. More usually, they were involved in a process of boundary creation and development. This meant that alongside any organisational rules, workers developed their own ideas about where and how boundaries should be made. A major feature of this chapter is its emphasis on boundary making as something that is both intuitive and learned. Through a discussion of how workers used a distinction between 'clients' and 'contacts' to help guide their behaviour, it is shown how boundary making also relied on pre-existing ideas about vulnerability, trust and power relationships.

Making boundaries

The idea that social work is involved in boundary making draws on Anselm Strauss' notion of deleted work (Strauss *et al.* 1985). This idea describes how the creation of structures and patterns of behaviour produces a sense of visible order in our life. However, the work needed to do this is often forgotten or 'deleted'. In order to understand how order is made we must search for deleted work. Within the context of this study, such a view implies that boundaries do not just exist, they are made. By implication, personal and professional spheres are shaped and constructed. It is important to look, therefore, at the work that goes into boundary making.

All of those interviewed felt they drew boundaries, and many spoke about this emphatically:

> *K:* So do you think boundaries are important?
>
> Oh they're absolutely kingpin really of a project working like this. I mean they're important (a) to protect the clients. They're also important to protect your project, and they're there also really for workers. (Edward, Midlands)

Many different kinds of boundaries were mentioned and this chapter focuses on the most commonly reported ones, rather than those that were idiosyncratic or individual. The boundaries most often referred to were those between sexuality and work, sex and work, home and work, leisure and work, and personal and professional feelings and behaviours. These were made in various ways through the use of statutory and organisational rules; supervision; different clothes, activities, places and times; distinctions between people; emotional control and mental focus; the control of information and self presentation.

It is important to note that different methods of boundary making were not necessarily separable and often interacted with one another. For example, boundaries between sex and work might be constructed using organisational rules, discussion of issues in supervision, by separating times for work and personal life, by seeking sexual partners in non-work places, by being wary of over sexualised self-presentation at work, and by making selective judgements about the types of people with whom it was appropriate to have sex.

Boundary development and understanding

More often than not, workers were involved in a process of boundary development. To some extent, this was the result of the relative newness of this type of outreach work at the time the study began, and the fact that agreed professional standards were still hotly debated. For those interviewed later, and those who were joining established projects, there was more likely to be an accepted organisational framework. However, even here people talked about organisational reviews of boundaries and described team discussions and developments that had changed their accepted practices and guidelines.

Not all workers had written organisational or project guidelines, and there were differences of opinion as to whether or not these were useful. However, regardless of whether or not rules had been codified, everyone felt a clear expectation from both their managers and organisations that boundary making was necessary.

Many outreach workers and their managers were fearful of the tabloid press,[1] and wanted to avoid public exposure of their work. Not surprisingly, the most heated discussion about boundaries therefore focused on prohibiting sex in certain circumstances. For example:

> We don't have sex with men from PSEs, or in the PSEs that we work in. We don't have sex with somebody we meet in a [commercial gay] venue on the day that we work that venue, or the evening after that … . We definitely don't have sex with anybody that we're involved in a counselling type relationship with … and we wouldn't have sex with anybody in all of these environments who we considered to be vulnerable … . And that's pretty much it. (Nick, London)

If a scandal occurred, being able to show the project had discussed the issues and operated within a clear code of conduct was felt to offer some protection. For this reason, written guidelines that workers could be shown to adhere to, were seen as a kind of insurance. As Rob explained, describing an occasion when, out of work, he had picked up a man in a PSE whom he later judged to be vulnerable, and therefore decided not to have sex with:

> I think if [as a project] we'd have said we're never going to have another boundary in our lives that would be ... that would make me feel quite edgy.
>
> *K:*   Right why would that be?
>
> Because I think, say the chap I picked up the other week. If things hadn't worked out well and I had to be very blatant and say: 'Well sorry I've decided I'm not going to have sex with you'. And then later on, a few months later ... he still feels quite badly about why I didn't have sex with him, and ... says well: 'Look, you know, I'm making a complaint about this, or I'm not happy about this'. Or, he starts telling other men he meets that ... we're just paid cock teasers, or stuff like that. Then I've nothing to fall back on ... . Whereas at the moment, I have something which I can turn around and quite confidently say: 'My professional judgement was that this person was in a vulnerable position' ... I'm sure that I would have the support [of my manager], and that you know his complaint ... would be met with, you know, a set of rules which are there to protect not only me, but him ... . No boundaries would have meant that, that would have been a very confusing and very messy event. (Rob, North)

Guidelines could also help workers communicate their responsibility and respectability when liaising with the police and other organisations. Making guidelines on boundaries known to others enabled these other professionals to distinguish when the workers were, and were not, undertaking outreach work. In this way they helped to communicate to both professionals and other gay men that the purpose of outreach work was not to make sexual contact, or seek sexual favours:

> Quite frequently the assumption is made by a lot of gay men who we talk to, that the reason we are in this job is because we want to be able to meet as many gay men as possible, in order to tap off and have sex ... . That's another reason why it's good to have these boundaries, and really stick to them, and really make them upfront. (Sean, North)

> You don't want them [other professionals] to misunderstand what's happening ... . You want them to value the work you're doing ... . If they think 'Oh you're just having sex' they're not going to take what you're really doing seriously ... . If I were out in my own social time, and I saw people that I knew, like other HIV workers, gay or lesbian project workers whatever, I would invariably say 'Hello' to them. But I'd also say 'Oh, you know, tonight's my night off' ... . It puts into their head the fact that sometimes you are working and sometimes you're not. So even if they don't come up and say 'Oh are you

working tonight?' it's like they see you chatting to someone, snogging some-one … then they would think 'Oh well, he must be surely not working'. (Isaac, Midlands)

The guidelines workers operated within varied according to their organisation, but covered issues such as maintaining confidentiality; not lending money or giving goods; not giving out a home telephone number; not having sex while working; not working under the influence of drugs; adhering to safety procedures; and not using work to meet personal needs. Sometimes, rules about behaviour were explicitly related to other codes of conduct. For example, alcohol consumption was often restricted to within the safe legal requirements for driving. In this way, project boundaries intersected with wider legal and statutory obligations.

Ownership

A major issue for workers was the importance of ownership over boundaries. Where workers had not been involved in developing guidelines, they were more likely to discuss having problems with them. It was stressed that organisations had to have 'manageable expectations' in which boundaries were agreed and workable rather than 'unrealistic' ones. Where working as part of a team, every-one needed to agree to, and adhere to, the guidelines. This was particularly impor-tant because workers would often draw on each other for support. Being able to be honest and discuss difficulties helped both to reinforce the idea of boundaries as professionally important and also to legitimise such issues as part of work. It also enabled workers to help each other when undertaking outreach work. For exam-ple, where co-workers had different views, talking helped them to negotiate a shared set of boundaries:

> We're a team that's very diverse. But at the same time you have a number of similar experiences, and you might have completely different viewpoints … but you've always [got] a debate and it's always easy to bring up issues around boundaries … in a really supportive [environment]. (Rob, North)

Discussions with others enabled boundary issues to be seen as a wider element of doing HIV prevention outreach work. This in turn helped their development and maintenance. For example, workers found it easier to work with men they were sexually attracted to, where they had thought and talked about this a lot as a team. This had prepared them to not act on sexual feelings.

> Talking with other workers really helps … . That feeling that you are not alone really, and you are not this sort of sex beast who really can't control his urges. Or, you are particularly unprofessional because you are feeling sexual towards people you are working with. (George, North)

For some men, these kinds of discussions were as important as written policies because they made boundaries part of an organisational process:

> I think having them [guidelines] is useful. But they have to be in existence with a kind of a process of how they're managed, and how they're instilled, how they're discussed and all that sort of stuff that goes with it ... . If you just have hard and fast guidelines and no kind of mechanisms for support or discussion that can actually be worse than having nothing at all. People just become really frightened by them and are less prepared to discuss, or consider even, any potential difficulties. (Alex, London)

An important part of this process involved support from managers. Workers felt supported by managers when they were able to talk about different strategies and discuss why boundaries had been a challenge or an issue. It was felt important, however, that such discussions took place with someone who appreciated the difficulties of outreach work.

The process of developing rules was seen to be very important. Some workers talked about having training and discussions around boundaries before agreeing them, and others talked about spending time coaching others about the need for them. However, this process was one of negotiation and dialogue, and was not necessarily straightforward:

> *K:* Maybe if you can just talk briefly about how they [organisational rules] came about?

> Yeah they came about through struggle ... . Fucking struggle, *(stamps foot)* ... I didn't at the time of bringing them in have a great feeling either way they should be there, they shouldn't be there. Um and I was speaking with [an experienced worker in the field]. And he was very clear and said: 'You've got boundaries. If they break them their sacked, they're out, it's no problem' *(slaps hand)* ... . So I brought that back into the project with an agenda to follow that ... . And the other aspect I raised, I think you have to have ownership of them. They're boundaries you are expected to keep to, and given they're such intensely personal things, you have to have ownership of how they are constructed and applied, in order that in reality they're something you work with rather than against ... . So, it was about team discussions what boundaries are we gonna have? And I was from the point of view no sex with anybody we meet in the work *(laughs)* ... that [was] my first point. And it was like 'aaahhh' *(horror from workers)* that's completely outrageous. And I think a lot of that was about: 'you're repressing my sexuality' ... . It took four weeks and a lot of sort of quite intense big discussions about why they should be there, the vulnerability of the men we work with, whether they are or aren't vulnerable and all these kinds of things, to eventually reach a point where we had a set that we agreed. (Nick, London)

Interestingly, Nick's account reveals a process of building on past experience and expertise as well as the idea of ownership. It also highlights an issue mentioned earlier, namely individual resistance to boundaries. Adhering to sexual codes of conduct has been an area in which gay men's workers report that they are being treated differently to others. This can make the process of boundary development difficult. For example, as Jill, an outreach manager, said:

> I asked the gay men if they'd like to set up a gay men's group about a year ago, to discuss this kind of issue. 'Cos I felt a bit uncomfortable sort of making policies around it when I don't know what it's like to use the cruising ground in my own time ... . There was me thinking for all these sort of PC [politically correct] reasons ... . They need to think about what boundaries they're comfortable with and advise us on making our policy, what we should do. And they were really angry *(laughs)*, that they'd been, that they were being focused on.(Jill, South)

The development of guidelines was commonly described as involving intense debates centring on identity politics and sexuality. Some workers would discuss the issue in terms of their right to have sex, but not everyone agreed with this. As Sarah said:

> I can't believe that there is an actual memo and people have been told that they're not to use the cruising sites. Surely that goes without saying? How come there's been so much time and energy that's gone into this whole thing around boundaries? ... . Obviously the gay man manager has to take on board the fact that there is a lot of unrest among the team, and it does need to be looked at ... . Like some people said they wanted to officially complain to the [Health] trust that there had been this ban imposed on them from using the [cruising] site 12 hours before and after [work], and how it infringed their life outside of work. And I think that's really dodgy ground ... . I don't think that cruising is a deviant activity, but I mean there is the law. (Sarah, London)

One way in which boundaries were developed was by using existing guidelines from other projects. This could occur both through talking to other outreach workers and reading literature. In addition, some workers built on guidelines from related areas of work, for example social work or counselling, although these rules often had to be adapted as they did not quite fit the nature of outreach work.

Above all, boundary making was a learning process. Workers had to learn to see the need for them, as well as how and when to implement them. Several people discussed using their own experiences of sexual abuse or burnout to inform their development of boundaries. In this way, they reported learning about the need for boundaries by going beyond or without them. Most commonly, it was suggested that the best learning about boundaries came through the experience of doing outreach work. Indeed, some workers suggested that they did not really get a handle on boundary issues until they had been doing the work for a while. Generally, making boundaries became easier over time as workers began to internalise their guidelines and moved towards a more intuitive style of boundary making. This was seen as a fluid process that was less about implementing a set of standard techniques, and more about developing a sense of judgement and what was often referred to as a 'work mentality' or an 'attitude to work'. It was this internalisation and intuitiveness that sometimes made it hard for people to articulate how exactly they drew boundaries:

> I'm sitting here thinking what do I do? And it's very difficult because you're actually out there thinking on your feet all the time. (Sandi, East)

It was noticeable that those interviewed later in the study tended to be much clearer about such issues. In part, this was perhaps because boundaries were being talked about among outreach workers generally on training courses and in articles in the gay press. However, it was also because this style of work was becoming more established. With the establishment of regional gay men's workers' forums in the UK in the mid-1990s, greater consistency began to emerge between projects as guidelines were more frequently shared, debated and discussed.

Flexibility

Not everyone had codified their boundary rules. One reason for this was a feeling that policies could not cover every eventuality and that by writing rules down procedures would become unnecessarily rigid. As a result, many workers sought a flexible framework in which they could use their own judgement. Although some felt that strict rules were better, as they led to less confusion, having guidelines that emphasised professional judgement was felt to give workers more freedom. However, not all boundaries were equally flexible, some were clearly non-negotiable and more important to maintain. For example:

> I don't do drugs, but if I did ... if somebody offered me drugs ... that's a non-flexible boundary. You know, as a prime example. But on the other aspect, if somebody meets me in the streets and I'm not working, and they ask me for a cup of tea, although we're not supposed to buy 'em one, I may buy 'em one. Because in the long run it may be better for the working, the professional relationship when I am working. (Derek, London)

> I mean I've always said to workers that I've supervised. Never lend anybody money. Ever. Any at all ... . Never take anybody home ... . You know if you wanna take somebody for coffee and buy them some chips I mean who cares? But it's getting into that kind of relationship that's very one sided [that's a problem]. I think really. (Tim, London)

Indeed in some organisations, most usually in the statutory sector, the breaking of certain boundaries was a dismissible offence.

The fact that many of the projects had decided to allow workers the flexibility to use their own judgement, albeit within a shared framework, meant that it was often left to individuals to develop their own strategies for boundary maintenance. This way of working meant that trust had to be developed between managers and workers:

> Well they [guidelines] were sort of vaguely written when I came into post and we've never seen a reason to tighten them up, because as I say [our manager] trusts sort of our common sense. (Roger, Midlands)

> I suppose that's where trust comes into work a lot, trusting the people you work with ... to undertake the work in a true and good faith. (Nick, London)

Given that outreach work usually took place beyond the direct gaze of management, workers had to take personal responsibility for boundary maintenance. The fact that the workers had few guidelines, had to make decisions on the hoof and often without the luxury of management advice meant that supervision was vital. As one person said: 'You deal with difficult situations there and then. Only if you choose to mention it, do others know [about your boundary issues].' As a result, there was a lot of pressure on individuals to be responsible in maintaining boundaries.

Clients, contacts and crumpet

Definitions and decisions concerning whom workers could and could not have sex with were central to establishing sexual boundaries. For some, this was quite clear:

> As a worker I shouldn't be having sex with people I come in contact with ... I'd even be cautious about having sex with other workers, let alone, service users. So no ... yeah ... I think I'm quite clear. (Craig, North)

> I've got very strict boundaries for me personally ... I wouldn't have sex with somebody that I work with in the same organisation, whatever level, volunteer, manager or director. I'd even think twice about having sex with somebody who does the same kind of work with another organisation. Because I think it becomes very complicated, especially in terms of HIV work, where it's a small network of people and they're all bonking away! *(laughs)* And I think it complicates things. (Nick, London)

However, others felt that defining who exactly was out of bounds was a complex process, particularly as the decision did not always reflect the desires of service users:

> But that brings up other issues about sort of like the rights of people, of like the clients as self-determined sexual people. Okay, they may have had a particular issue at one point in their life, [but] what happens maybe when they have worked through that ... . And, you know they wanted to have sex with you, and maybe you wanted to have sex with them? It feels like quite patronising to

say … that we are always going to be in this powerful position over you … . And if ever we slept with you it's because we're going to be abusing you. (George, North)

One of the reasons why workers reported finding boundary making hard was that they did not have a clear client-type relationship with every individual they worked with. This meant they had to make judgements on the hoof. The boundaries that different workers and organisations operated within differed, but most seemed to distinguish between users with whom they had had a more involved or long-term working relationship and more superficial 'contacts'. The understanding was that when they were not working workers could have sex with contacts but 'clients' were out of bounds in relation to sexual contact:

I sort of say, well if I've given somebody a condom in the middle of a nightclub then it's okay to go off with them. If I've had, I don't know, a counselling session for instance with somebody else then, then that's not all right. (Richard, Midlands)

Many workers suggested that these distinctions would always be open to interpretation and that inevitably no definitive guideline could be made. There were, however, certain characteristics that people used to help them decide who was 'out of bounds':

Obviously there were like the clear ones, like the people who are in the [support] groups, and people that we'd talked to face to face, or on the telephone. The grey areas are people like volunteers, for example, and we decided that no, we shouldn't sleep with people who are volunteers either … . You've just got to use your common sense … . If they're kind of like, confident, out [about their sexuality], with a network of friends, then I think it's fine to sleep with them. (Sean, North)

If I went and did like a workshop at a youth group, I wouldn't have sex with one of the men in the workshop … . If I was to give a talk at [a voluntary group] and it was all these really assertive gay men that I partly knew anyway, I wouldn't have a problem with having sex with one of them afterwards. But if it was a coming out group … and it was some man who happened to be 35 but was obviously quite insecure, I just wouldn't. (Jason, London)

Figure 3 on page 112 shows the main features workers used to differentiate between contacts and clients.

Importantly, underlying these distinctions was the idea of power. For example, in response to the question: 'How would you go about defining who's a client?', workers replied:

I'd use that power definition. How much someone's disclosed to you … . Whether they've come to you, or you've come to them in some ways. But also

Contact	Client
Brief contact	Lengthy contact
Superficial chat	In-depth discussion
One-off contact	Ongoing relationship
Handed a condom	Given counselling
Small amount of information disclosed	Large amount of information disclosed
Seeking general information	Has an identifiable problem
Needs practical help	
Fancy them; good looking	Don't want sex with; can't have sex with
Peer	Clear power differential
You've approached them	They've approached you
Used your knowledge/skills	
Seeking support	
Confident	Vulnerable

Figure 3 Distinctions between contacts and clients.

whether they've looked at you as a professional, and used your knowledge, skills as a professional. But I think the core thing is the power thing. (Toby, North)

I guess it would be somebody who, you're there to deliver a service to, and in some ways delivering that service means that you are able to influence them somehow. (Tim, London)

In the broader counselling literature, issues of power are explicitly discussed in relation to sexual relationships with clients. There is an emphasis on the importance of maintaining a therapeutic trusting relationship through establishing professional boundaries with clients. However, in outreach work where workers had many different types of relationship with men, rather than making generalised statements about the types of people who should be classed as clients, most workers said their organisations allowed them to use 'professional judgement'. Decisions were made on individual cases using the kinds of characteristics outlined in Figure 3.

Places and spaces

As noted in the previous chapter, some of the most common organisational guidelines related to place. Where possible, workers established boundaries by using
different places to have sex, meet sexual partners and socialise, to the places in
which they worked. This was a strategy that was discussed, even if not used, by
all. For example, in the first ten interviews conducted, all the workers said they
would not use the public sex environments where they worked for their own purposes, and some would not socialise in the same clubs where they worked. Later
in the research, however, workers talked about developing more sophisticated
sexual boundary rules related to the various venues where they worked:

> It's about different boundaries for different pieces of work. And so the work
> we do in venues, our boundaries aren't as strict [as in PSEs] … . We wouldn't
> have sex in the venue, or go away with somebody from that venue and have
> sex on the same night, or the same day. But we're entitled to exchange phone
> numbers, or at least make the fact that sex might go on an issue, and plan for
> that. (Nick, London)

It is interesting to note that sexual boundaries were often established in relation
to existing spatial boundaries: for example, the borders of health authorities or the
towns in which outreach work occurred. Some workers made boundaries by refus-
ing to work in certain areas or restricted the places where they worked, to ensure
that they had alternative places in which to socialise or seek sex:

> As far as it's possible, I try not now to socialise around the area that I work, in
> terms of like pubs and clubs, that I always try and go out of the area. (Richard,
> Midlands)

> I have boundaries around … where I socialise in the context of where I geo-
> graphically work. I don't tend to socialise in the area, [the] geographical area
> that I work in. And I wouldn't use those PSEs … in the area that I work in.
> (Nick, London)

As described earlier, for some this form of boundary making was difficult. For
example, if there was only one gay club in the locality then workers had to socialise and meet potential sexual partners where they worked, unless they could afford
to travel to another town. For those who socialised outside the commercial gay
scene boundaries were already constituted in terms of place. Having different
places in which to socialise meant that these workers had access to an alternative
space that was clearly separate from work, one in which they did not have to think
about their role as a service provider. This use of different kinds of place was discussed in terms of enabling people to feel different to when they were at work.

In a contrasting but possibly related way, those in monogamous long-term sexual
relationships frequently mentioned that this helped them to draw boundaries;[2] not

only did they have a life which they saw as separate from work, but also they did not have to deal with a lot of potentially confusing issues: such as using the places they worked in to find sexual partners.

Many workers tried to maintain a distinction between home and work life even though they recognised that crossovers were inevitable. In this way, the use of different places was a convenient and visible form of boundary making. People would socialise elsewhere, use straight pubs, and go away for weekends or breaks in different towns. Others would cultivate their personal space, with home becoming an important space of sanctuary:

> Sometimes I'll say to myself right I've had, I can't cope with whatever is going on and I tell everybody I'm going away for the weekend. Sometimes I do, sometimes I just stay here! And I have 48 hours in my own home, with only a few, a handful of people knowing where I am. Where I can indulge in um … I dunno my science fiction books, I can watch the television, have a few beers and forget completely about HIV and AIDS. (Sandi, East)

> I think I spend more time just switching off totally and sitting in my flat than I probably would if I was doing an office job. It's a different, different kind of relief about getting home. In fact going to the pub for a drink might be more stressful than it is to sit at home! *(laughs)* Yeah? (Toby, North)

Place in work

Boundaries were also drawn within work. This might involve not working in the most sexualised areas of clubs or cruising grounds. For example, Rob said he had stopped going to the parts of the cruising area where: 'People would get their dicks out while you were talking to them and wank.' He worked instead in areas where people were more willing to engage in conversation:

> You walk around only part of the area, and you don't enter into dense undergrowth or various paths which are dead ends and you keep on a circuit … . If I'm cruising myself then I'm more likely to start tempting people by walking up the dead ended paths or, or going into bushes and stuff. And you know by doing that you're sort of saying to them 'Hey let's go and have some sex'. I think when you're working you're, you're blending in by being there and by looking cruisy … but not to the same extent … . You're only being in safe areas. In the open areas. You're in the sort of meeting areas; you're not going into any of the doing places. If you do, it's usually with your co-worker, and it's usually to leave some condoms there, or you know just to look for evidence that people are still having sex there. (Rob, North)

A further way in which the use of space was used to maintain boundaries occurred when workers deliberately withdrew from a situation. In this respect, having guidelines that encouraged thought about personal safety was important. However, keeping boundaries by exiting a space was usually seen as a last resort:

> You'll always get the persistent ones [clients], often they're drunk so *(laughs)* .... Then it is about having to leave the site ... I can only think of once in two years now where somebody's followed me off site, but fortunately we'd got the car and we just got in the car and drove off. (Derek, London)

Times

When workers used the same places for work and socialising, time could be used to demarcate purpose and intent. Some workers, for example, used venues for socialising at times, or on days, different to when they worked. A few projects had decided that workers could use venues where they undertook outreach work for personal reasons as soon as a session had ended. Several workers felt that this was not a good idea since sudden changes could be potentially confusing for all concerned:

> If you're saying to somebody: 'Oh come back at the end of the night', or 'I'm going to be here on Saturday come back then', I mean you may as well say 'Yes' there and then. As far as I'm concerned, you're still picking them up while you're working .... Or that's how I see it anyway. So I think that's a bit dodgy personally. (Craig, North)

> I think that that is really taking the piss if you like. Because sort of, for two hours you're there, and you're telling men that you're there to talk about HIV and AIDS, sexual health, talk about all those various issues. And then ten minutes later you go there and go 'OK wop your cock out then' .... That I think is sending out very disturbing messages. Um ... and messages which I believe for me could get you into very sticky situations .... Especially [when] some of the men that we meet, or are likely to meet, you know, as soon as you appear on the scene they drop their trousers, they start wanking and if that's going to happen then it can get you into all sorts of hassles .... For me that is playing with people and so that's something I wouldn't encourage. (Rob, North)

Professional responsibility was seen as an enduring commitment by some interviewees:

> I mean, I can see what people are doing but .... Well I just kind of think you're a worker .... You know, if you're a doctor and you meet your patient out in the street then somehow just 'cos you're not in the waiting room doesn't mean that you don't have professional responsibilities and professional ethics to uphold you know. Or a counsellor and a client who by chance meet at the same party. It doesn't mean that they don't have that relationship .... It's like trying to trick the boundary *(laughs)*. (Tim, London)

Another way in which time was used to create boundaries was through limiting interactions with clients. For example, when working outreach workers would try to contact as many people as possible, rather than just talking to one person, as they might do when they were socialising. This was one way in which they tried to ensure that there was equitable service delivery. However, the focus and content of the interaction sometimes affected boundary making here:

> If, for example, a guy told us that he'd been raped two nights before, then that's the sort of conversation that I'd allow to go on all night. But if it's some-body just waffling on about his partners, and all these different partners he's had then … there's no benefit for myself as a worker in it. What information can I give this person? Because at the end of the day that's what I'm there for. I'm there to give information and materials and only get minimal information back. So if there's nothing in it for me then it is about, 'We'll maybe we'll see you later'. (Derek, London)

This example highlights the way in which professional judgements often had to be made in interpreting guidelines. Boundaries would be made or broken in ways that were tailored to the context and individual. In this way, boundary making was very much an interactive process.

Clothing

Just under half the workers talked in detail about how clothing was used to help establish boundaries between work and non-work. In club and pub work, special project T-shirts might be worn, for example, although people also mentioned project bomber jackets and wearing accessories such as badges or ID. These clothes and accessories were used to signal to themselves, and others, when they were and were not working:

> I mean if I'm in a T-shirt I'm working. (Toby, North)

> People generally know that unless … they see us with our T-shirts on that … we're *not* working. So we always carry a change of clothes. We always put the badges away. We always, you know we try and look as differently as possible to when we're working. (Edward, Midlands)

Those who found this strategy helpful felt that specific clothes provided a useful visual marker:

> [Wearing T-shirts helps] because it gives us an identity, we're recognisable. We're somewhat approachable, like a uniform yeah … . It helps more for our-selves to give us confidence, because it gives a sort of a reason for being there and reminds us that we're working. (Andrew, North)

And there are rules and regulations for [the organisation] that while they've got that T-shirt on they're working … . They gotta get rid of the T-shirt before they start socialising. So it's almost like coming out from behind a counter. That makes it much more definable. (Sandi, East)

It is revealing that phrases such as 'having a uniform' and 'coming out from the counter' were used by workers as these signal a link with other professionals and service industries. The use of different clothes is a technique drawn upon in many other occupations. For example, Hochschild (1983) reports that Delta Airlines would not allow employees to enter a bar or drink while in uniform and that American Airlines would not allow short sleeved shirts as they 'lacked authority'. Macdonald on the other hand describes how accountants often have strict dress codes which he reports include the allowing of grey or blue suits, not brown, and no facial hair (1995). He argues that the use of clothes is a way in which professionals' knowledge and trustworthiness is signalled (see also Paterson 1983). In this way, getting changed after work gives a visible signal to oneself and others about a shift in role.

To work as a boundary, the symbolic nature of work and non-work clothes had to be accepted and noticed by service users, who have to be educated about the symbolic value of appearance. Although the meaning of particular symbols was often obvious to workers, this was not necessarily the case for others. Where workers did not have project uniforms, or men were not aware of the project, difficulties were caused by not having the usual accoutrements to signal that they were at work. For example:

I think sometimes people do have difficulty understanding that you really are working, even if you've said it and they've heard you. Because, you know, people don't have this idea that you go to a social venue to work. Unless you were to walk around with a clipper board or something and then they could at least say 'Oh well he's doing a survey in clubs about you know gay men'. But if you just look like anyone [it's difficult]. (Isaac, Midlands)

Not all men are going to even have an understanding of the work, of the issues, of anything really apart from a blowjob. Some of them, when you're talking to them that's the only thing they can see … . What they're there for is that blowjob and that's it. And they'll do anything to get that. (Rob, North)

This again highlights the interactive nature of successful boundary making. For those working in small towns, people quickly adapted to well known symbols such as T-shirts and began to understand their significance, learning when they could and could not approach the workers. In this way people would modify their own behaviour so as to help maintain the boundaries workers had created.

Some workers gave a lot of thought to the clothes they wore in order to help establish the right relationship with contacts, clients and other professionals. As Sarah (London) said, describing her clothes for outreach work:

> I suppose your clothes are really important, because you wouldn't go wearing a power suit when you're working with the homeless. You wouldn't have anything that could be intimidating … . We are at the end of the day outreach workers and it's for us to get on other people's territories and get to know them in their environment … . I think people have got big things around their self-esteem, especially homeless people, or rent boys, or people like that … . And I think if you try and like show that you're really in love with yourself by having sort of wonderful clothes and a full face of make-up I don't think that's relating very well to your sort of client group. (Sarah, London)

Other workers chose not to wear certain kinds of clothes when in the office: for example, T-shirts with slogans that were political or related to gay issues. However, others purposefully pushed boundaries in this manner, especially if they wanted to make a statement about their sexuality, or challenge organisational homophobia as described in Chapter 4:

> I tend to play up when it comes to clothes … my predecessor had big arguments about wearing jeans … the Health Care Trust thought this broke their boundaries and they just could not accept the situation. And the previous worker claimed it was part of gay culture and heritage, which I thought was fabulous! And so far from let that lapse I've most probably played up to it. And I can be fairly outrageous if I want to be in what I wear. (Steve, North)

Interestingly, issues of 'appropriate dress' have at times proved inflammatory in AIDS organisations (Carter 1995; Phoenix 1995) and highlight potential conflicts between gay and professional identities.

Presentation: making roles clear

Different forms of self-presentation were also crucial in developing and maintaining boundaries. For example, people said that when doing outreach work, it was important to think about the way they spoke, looked and acted and what these forms of behaviour suggested to others. Above all, when working many stressed that they would not follow up or play up to sexual interest:

> I mean a lot of men will be very persistent in cruising you … . But I think to give any indication that you might be interested in them is wrong if you're going to turn around and say: 'We're employed by the health authority, and here's your safer sex pack but you're not going to use it with me'. (Bill, Midlands)

> You can't afford I think to be as blatant sometimes as I am when I'm cruising in my own time, because you don't want to lead people on too much. So that, you know, they're convinced that you're going to have sex with them no matter what. (Rob, North)

Workers also had to think about how they reacted to body language themselves, especially unwanted proximity or touch:

> It is really awful when you've got someone sort of breathing beer fumes down your neck and occasionally they won't take no for an answer, and [you] need to be sort of really firm with them. Sort of threaten them with the bouncers or whatever. And they do back down, but you have to be sort of quite strong-minded to stop it getting out of hand. (Roger, Midlands)

> A man in the pub had chatted to me briefly earlier; we'd talked about the role of [the project], why we were there to give out condoms, etc. etc. He'd noticed that I was quite hairy as a person, and yanked my T-shirt to have a look at my chest hair. Um ... you know, it was a little bit close to the mark, but I can deal with that. That's not a ... gross invasion as far as I'm concerned. But then later on in the evening when I went around the pub distributing condoms, trying to be a bit more proactive ... he actually grabbed me by the crotch. At which point I just put my hand up and pushed him away, quite firmly said: 'Look, you know, this is not on. I'm not here for this'. (Steve, North)

In general, workers felt that it was best to have little or no physical contact with service users. In this way boundaries were made through setting limits on physical interaction. However, the interactive nature of sexual encounters meant that boundaries were not always completely within workers' control. For example, as Tim said when describing what behaviour he considered out of bounds:

> Well I would say anything beyond a bit of jokey flirting really *(laughs)* ... . But that's tricky. I mean that is really tricky because I've worked with ... young men with learning difficulties who, when I was explaining safer sex to them, and my boundaries were really clear, I was not kind of doing anything untoward, they got stiffies. (Tim, London)

Workers found that it was useful to make their role clear early on, to prevent any confusion. This was particularly so in PSE work where it would be logical for the men they were working with to assume they were there to have sex, or were the police:

> When you make the initial contact it's very important to actually say: 'Look I'm not here for the purposes that you think I am', or 'I don't want to waste your time', 'cos you know people are on the way home from work or something and they haven't got time to waste and you're invading their privacy essentially. So, it's very important to say ... 'These are the services we can provide you, do you need condoms, do you need lubricant, have you got any particular questions that you think we can help you with?' (Roger, Midlands)

Some people will leap out of the bushes with something hanging out from their trousers and my thing then is: 'I'm not here for sex, my name is X and I'm a health education worker, and I'm here to talk about health issues around gay sex.' (Sandi, East)

As highlighted earlier, boundary making could also be difficult because service users did not always recognise, or appreciate, workers' different roles. While most men accepted the idea of professional boundaries, a few were more difficult.[3] For example, some men accepted that there could be no sex at that time, but expected workers would have sex with them afterwards. Very occasionally men would be angry that they had been led on:

Occasionally people will be pissed off, and will show that and stop communicating with you ... that's fairly rare. Some people will push even further once you've asserted the boundary ... . Some people will respect it and that's fine and then the communication will continue. And I think some people probably just don't believe it and, and constantly re-engage on that level ... . The majority of times I would say people either respect it, or they'd pull back and are probably a little bit confused by it. (Nick, London)

Workers had to put a lot of effort into explaining boundaries in a way that made sense to others and communicated their role. Asserting boundaries required skill because workers had to ensure that they maintained good working relationships; too hasty a reaction could make it difficult to enter a site or venue again. An important consideration was to ensure that people did not feel rejected by the way boundaries were introduced:

What I think is important is that we're affirmative in the way we do it ... . My standard one is: 'I think you're really attractive but I don't fancy you!' *(laughs)*. Which, I mean it could be a complete lie because I might not think they're attractive at all ... I don't feel completely comfortable about lying, but I think it's a really important thing just to say to someone that they are attractive, whether you personally find them attractive or not *(laughs)*. Um ... just because of men feeling quite low. And men quite often talk about how, oh you know, 'No one gets off with me' sort of thing. (Toby, North)

Several people mentioned the use of humour to help draw boundaries. When working in clubs, this strategy was used quite frequently because it fitted the social context, perhaps in the way barmaids sometimes use put-downs to stop sexual innuendo:

K: What about the groping and things like that, how do you deal with it?

Well I, it's all that sort of very, you know 'Don't touch what you can't afford' and all that. I never really challenge it in a serious way. It's always been like on a very clubby sort of way ... . It's all that jokey 'not now' and all that, and going into the banter really ... . Sometimes, I just feel like smacking some-body in the face and saying you know 'Don't think I'm a vacuous blonde bimbo' you know. (George, North)

Some workers suggested that being humorous diffused the tension in potentially difficult situations. Again, the context and the nature of the individual involved was a factor to be taken into account, as Jill recounts:

I had a gay man really sort of grabbed my bum on the van and squeezed it, you know. And he was doing it to the gay men as well ... . He was drunk ... . And I think I dealt with that with humour, in that I said something like 'I think you're a bit confused darling! Just grabbed the wrong variety of bottom!', or some-thing ... . But then we had another client ... who I find very threatening. He never takes his motorbike helmet off, and he smells *(laughs)* ... . He came and sat next to me, and he sat really close and he was talking to me and he tried to touch my face, to do that *(pinches)* on my cheek. And he went to touch me and I said 'Don't touch me'. And I was deadly serious with him because I don't like him. I find him threatening ... . He was saying 'Oh I was only going to pinch your cheek'. I said 'Well yes I know what you were going to do' I said, 'But what I'm saying is I don't want you to touch me like that at all, OK?' And he sort of went 'Right OK', you know just carried on talking or whatever was going on ... . So I would tend to use humour to deal with most situations, unless I feel very insecure. (Jill, South)

In outreach situations boundaries were often continually being tested and negoti-ated. For example, men might be sexually excited, drunk or simply not really take in what was being said. This meant that workers had constantly to be on their guard:

I mean, every time he meets me he always asks me whether he can fuck me and you go 'No', and he says 'Why not?', and you go 'Well, because you can't'. And that's difficult. So every single time he says 'Can I fuck you, can I fuck you, when are you going to fuck me?' ... . That's just one of the problems of the job. Because you are giving off sexual signals, you're working in a sexual environment and it would be unrealistic not to expect people to respond to those. (Andrew, North)

One of the strategies used to facilitate boundary making was to tell men about their guidelines or make references to similar situations. For example, by drawing parallels with men's own occupations.

Psychological boundaries

Another method workers used to separate themselves from their work involved drawing boundaries 'psychologically'. This was felt to be important because of the lack of visible barriers in outreach work:

> I think that's probably one of the greatest difficulties really ... how compara-
> tively barrierless it is. I mean, even on a basic level working in an office you
> have control about who comes through the door you know. And you don't on
> the street, or you don't in a club. People come up to you. And also you know
> those barriers are real like your desk is a real physical barrier and you don't
> have that on the [street] ... . And so there maybe have to be psychological
> boundaries. (George, North)

Such boundaries offered a form of professional detachment that enabled workers to focus on service provision. Interviewees said that they tried to divorce themselves from their feelings, tried not to get emotionally involved or sexually aroused
by what was being said to them, and focused on the best methods of service provision. The use of such psychological techniques was described by some as a form of
disciplining:

> I find it easier to handle gay clubs and the scene when I'm there to work than I
> do when I'm there socially, strangely. Because I've got a reason for being
> there, and a set of guidelines to follow, and I know how to behave. (Sean,
> North)

> I think it's also an attitude to work, because it's about when you are working,
> saying: 'I am working and I am not there to further anything personal, and I'm
> clearly in this role now'. (Toby, North)

This psychological orientation was talked about using phrases such as 'work
mentality'; 'in my mind'; 'worker mode'; 'thing at the back of your mind'; 'attitude to work'. Some felt that this clear work focus lay at the core of boundary
making. Being clear in your own mind about boundaries made it easier both to
communicate them to others (Rosica 1995, Ussher 1993) and also to maintain
boundaries in various situations. This work focus also enabled workers to remain
non-judgmental and concentrate on the needs of the men they contacted.

Self-disclosure

Finally, boundaries were created by workers controlling personal information
about themselves. This was an area where there were quite a few differing views
as to what should be done. Some felt it was important to share personal information in order to build trust:

> I will tell people about my private life to the extent where it will facilitate what
> I'm trying to do. I never give my home phone number; I never give my address
> out. But I would tell 'em that I live in Green Town ... . Because if somebody
> lives out [Green Town] way, that's where they're brought up, by my saying
> 'Oh I live out [Green Town] way', then automatic they've got a link. Some-
> thing they can hook into. And that's what it's about. (Derek, London)

Others, however, felt that it was inappropriate to provide personal information:

> The way you talk about things is quite important. I mean, not in a clinical way, but to make sure you don't use personal experience to explain things to people. You don't say 'Well I do this, I do that' because ... that I think is breaking those personal boundaries. Because the job is not about what I do, and what I don't do, it's a more generalised thing ... I would try and make them relate their experiences to what I was trying to tell them, rather than me relating my experience to them. And that draws a kind of personal boundary. (Sean, North)

However, as Sean went on to say, the content of the interaction affected the way he would use these techniques:

> It varies from situation to situation. I mean, if I was talking to somebody about say a specific sexual practice and they said. Quite frequently people say, 'Oh what do you do in that situation? ... Have you ever fucked without a condom?' and stuff like that. And I might say, 'Yes I have'. But then I try and steer the conversation away from what I do, and what I'm not doing. (Sean, North)

As well as controlling personal information about themselves, some workers established boundaries by hiding the feelings they may have had towards clients. This was particularly the case with people they found annoying or when they were challenged by men they approached:

> And also you need to be aware that ... they might tell you to fuck off. Or they might say 'What do you think I'm doing here?' you know, 'Do you think I'm sick or something?' When you know they've just gone in there, into the urinals to try to suck someone off. And yet they're still going to come out with stuff about 'Well I'm not queer' and sort of homophobic stuff. And you just have to accept that. You can't go and challenge everyone. (Andrew, North)

Analysing and controlling personal emotions was an important way of ensuring that boundaries were maintained. Workers discussed using supervision and talking with colleagues as a way of venting their anger or negative feelings. The use of supervision encouraged interviewees to look at their own reactions in order to learn to manage their boundaries more effectively, for example, through developing skills to recognise where their personal difficulties or interests affected the way they worked:

> A lot of people in this work go into their own therapy right in order to become more self aware, so that they can check some of the things they're doing in their jobs. (Erkan, London)

Before a session, we always talk about how we're feeling. You always sort of try and analyse, and try and be self aware of how you're feeling … . And we know how our partner's feeling as well … . It just helps you read situations better in the end. (Edward, Midlands)

Supervision and other kinds of support were vital in enabling workers to look after themselves emotionally. This was crucial in such person centred work:

I think you need to have a certain amount of armour as protection as a worker. Because you're constantly hearing stories of abuse and tales of, I don't know, you do get to hear so much negative stuff … . And by having those boundaries people don't get into you too much … I think giving more than you are able to cope with is abusive to yourself, and also to your client group. (Sarah, London)

As de Croy (1990) writes:

Outreach work succeeds or fails on the ability to interact sensitively and effectively with men who have sex with men, and therefore the key tool a worker has is their own personality. Because of this, workers looking after themselves emotionally is not a side issue, but is central to the work being effective.

(de Croy 1990:28)

Although workers could value support from colleagues, some were scared to discuss boundary issues with them. One of the reasons given for this was that as men they found it hard to talk about feelings. This difficulty has been noted elsewhere as being linked to dominant ideologies and expectations of masculinity. Victor Seidler (1991) writes:

Our first response as men is often to deny whatever we are feeling, because the very fact that we are feeling anything is taken as a sign that we are not 'in control'. So it becomes difficult to legitimate whatever feelings we have, especially at work – where we can fear being exposed and ridiculed by other men.

(Seidler 1991:127)

And as Nick explained, there was often a macho culture in team meetings:

There seems to be a general thing about outreach … working on the streets it's like: 'Hey I'm totally cool and I'm there, and you know I can look after myself'. And that is all about machismo. And that environment tends to work against people being able to examine them [boundaries], explore them properly. (Nick, London)

Nick further suggested that to have issues around boundaries suggested vulnerability, whereas other gay men expected him to have sexual prowess and confidence.

The difficulty in discussing feelings meant that seeking support around boundary issues was hard for some, and workers were often choosy about whom they shared personal information with. Indeed, although some felt that it was useful to talk to their partners about work in order to get support, others agreed not to talk about work at home in order to maintain a sense of boundaries.

Conclusions

Overall, boundary making was a continual learning process in which guidelines were subject to change and negotiation and were adapted over time. Even where there were formal guidelines these always had to be interpreted, which meant that workers had to learn how to understand and apply the rules. The development of boundaries helped workers to manage the various tensions created by their occupational role. For example, using sexual signals to make contact with service users but not actually having sex whilst working, or building trust without relying too much on personal experience. In order to give workers the flexibility to adapt boundaries to suit different contexts and needs, they were often written in a way that encouraged the use of intuition and judgement. In this way, boundary making involved developing a sense of judgement and an 'attitude to work' rather than the implementation of a set of standard techniques.

It was clear that the meaning of workers' roles and associated boundaries were negotiated through their interaction with service users, managers and organisations. This meant that boundaries could also be resisted or challenged by others, or that other people might help in their maintenance. Because of the nature of their working environment, a lot of boundary work involved managing their own, and others', emotions and expectations. Workers had to educate others in the symbolic ways in which they drew boundaries.

7 Professionalism and sexual identity

One of the main ways in which workers constructed boundaries within work, and between work and other parts of their life, was through internalised ideas about 'being professional'. There were several ways in which the idea of professionalism was expressed in boundary making. One of the most obvious was in its articulation through organisational guidelines: such rules provided workers with a framework to guide professional conduct and enforced ideas about acceptable behaviour. In fact the need to be seen to 'be professional' was one of the main reasons given for having boundaries and workers stated that they were continually told by their managers to draw boundaries in order to be professional:

> I know that I have to have boundaries because I am a professional in that sense. (Sanjay, East)

> [Boundaries are] about being effective, about I'd say professional ... about delivering quality and effective services. (Nick, London)

Despite the emphasis many placed on 'being professional', the relationship between professionalism and sexual identity raised numerous tensions and issues. In fact, workers had very different feelings about this relationship:

> This one I feel I have difficulty with. I've seen people who are in similar jobs and they have very different titles: 'Senior health promotion specialist for gay men'. What does that mean? What would that say to people? ... . That sounds as if it's, you know, I'm up here, everyone else is down there. That I'm a professional first and foremost, and only a gay man by chance. I think when you over-professionalise this area of work, you run into a problem where ... you distance yourself from the grassroots. And in particular in this project, it's community development, we're supposed to be grassroots and bottom up led. Then, you know, calling yourself a professional constantly is not aiding that process at all.
>
> *K:* Because it's creating a sort of power difference or ... ?
>
> Yeah, and knowledge difference and everything really. You know, calling

yourself a health professional ... puts you on a level with a doctor or, it puts you well above what you are actually doing. And I think that can only be negative. (Rob, North)

Professionalism is really important to me, and I think more than anything my heart is with a kind of generation of, of gay male professionals who have expertise in sexual health ... I want there to be a body of highly professionalised, actually, highly professionalised gay men with expertise in this field. I think there should be ... . And that doesn't mean I don't believe in volunteerism or political activism ... [but] I'm really very taken by the notion of a whole body of knowledge and a whole body of expertise and a whole body of practice existing now where it didn't ten years ago. I find that very captivating somehow. And very inspiring. So I believe in professionalism more than anything. (Tim, London)

Professionalism, sex and sexuality

In many ways, dominant ideas of 'being professional' can be seen to exclude sex and sexuality. This separation can be seen in the way that many people working in the field of sexuality have experienced difficulties in getting their work taken seriously (see for example Allgeier 1984; Fisher 1989; Hart 1992; Lindenbaum 1991 and Udry 1993;), or have experienced ridicule and abuse. Similarly, those who have attempted to address issues relating to sexual boundaries within their professions have often found it impossible to conduct (Brodsky 1989), or report on their research (Rutter 1991), or have faced hostility for daring to address the issue (Gechtman 1989). Since sex has often been disregarded as a legitimate work topic it is perhaps not surprising that issues pertaining to sex and sexuality have been difficult to validate as professional concerns.

There is clearly a sense, therefore, in which the professional and the sexual are seen as excluding each other. This also applies to HIV prevention outreach work. For example, even though the work involves discussing issues of sex and sexuality, working in sexualised environments, and being open about their own sexuality, many workers still found it hard to talk about boundary issues with management for fear of being labelled unprofessional:

I don't think I would feel able to go to the board of management and say: 'Look I slept with someone who may be construed as a client' ... I just don't think I'd be able to do that ... I think that would be a major knock really, I think, to how people would perceive my professionalism. (George, North)

You see we're always trying to be professional. And this is what we're always being told. You know, 'You must be professional'. Which is fair enough, I mean obviously that needs to be so. But it's like sometimes, you know, if you fancy someone, or something that might have come close to something that shouldn't have happened ... . Do you really want to say [so], because what will people think? (Isaac, East)

In some professions there has long been an imperative not to have sex with clients. For example, this is true of doctors (Dillner 1996), and Abramson (1992) mentions it in relation to ethnographic research. More recently, some professions have codified this proscription, with guidelines concerning sexual conduct being developed for the clergy (Thomas 1995), sex researchers (Society for the Scientific Study of Sex 1993) and lecturers (Brookman 1993; MacLeod 1993; Maslen 1995; Meikle 1992; *Times Higher Educational Supplement* 1995). Therefore, it is perhaps unsurprising that most of the workers had a clause built into their code of conduct relating to not having sex with clients. Such proscriptions have a long history as Brodsky notes:

> References to the issue of sex between therapist and patient date back to the Hippocratic oath, which warns physicians not to have sex with their patients, and further back to statements in the code of the Nigerian medicine men, who were advised not to 'sex the patient'.
>
> (Brodsky 1989:15)

However, it was not until the mid-1970s that patient–therapist sex was clearly declared unethical by the US mental health professions (later being made illegal in some states), and only in 1980 was it written into USA social work codes. Given the lack of formal guidelines relating to sexual contact in many organisations, outreach workers' codes of conduct could be seen as surprising.

Views of sex, sexuality and professionalism as entirely separate are both problematic and contradictory, as professionalism and sex can also be seen to be intertwined. For example, being a 'professional' and 'the oldest profession' are both euphemisms for prostitution. Furthermore, (tabloid) newspapers frequently sensationalise the 'sexual antics' of professionals such as judges, doctors and priests (Bedell 1991; Gledhill 1996; Grant 1992). Although part of the shock value here derives from the bringing together of things that are supposed to be separate, such revelations highlight the fact that sex and work are linked, for example through love affairs, sexual exploits on business trips and sexual harassment. Moreover, as noted in Chapter 1, recent sociological and psychological research has begun to reveal connections between sexuality and professionalism in the growing literatures on organisational sexuality, and sexual relationships between professionals and their different types of clients.

Professionalism in the context of gay and bisexual men's HIV prevention

Outreach workers employed notions of professional behaviour in various ways. Work with gay and bisexual men takes place in a broader political and cultural climate that is not favourable. For workers, there is always the possibility of a local scandal that could stop the work; therefore they felt the need to present a respectable image:

> Because the work is very new, and because of its highly sexual nature, and because of its titillating sort of bits to it. Unless we are seen I think as acting in the upmost *(sic)* professionalism, then the work will be undervalued completely and people will see us as, you know, as a couple of gay boys having a good time. (George, North)

The perceived importance of boundaries lay in their ability to ensure that HIV prevention workers were seen as providing a professional service. Importantly, however, many gay men were interested not only in protecting the work because of a concern for professionalism, but also because of a personal responsibility to the wider community:

> We are all very protective of the project and we really wouldn't intentionally do anything that would bring the project into disrepute. 'Cos there's so little being done for gay men, you've got to protect what there is. And we are all gay men after all. So we're protecting our own interests as well as those of our client group. (Roger, Midlands)

By 'being professional', workers felt that they could both gain acceptance for their work and be taken seriously by other professionals. The fact that they were being paid to undertake the work they did was seen as of great importance in this respect. Being paid was felt to change the relationship workers had with other gay men. As paid service providers, most thought that they should be aware of their position and the responsibilities it carried. Payment established a particular relationship not only with service users, but also with the employer. For this reason, it was argued that volunteers faced different boundary issues to paid workers. Some suggested that volunteers had less responsibility and less to lose, as they did not have the same public accountability.

The pressure to compete for funds was a powerful professionalising influence, and workers tried hard to appear professional to communicate the importance of the work. This involved demonstrating that outreach work was much more demanding than 'just hanging around with gay men in clubs', or 'being paid to go cruising':

> It's not just about going to a pub once a week and, you know, spending six hours a week outside a cottage. It's about having things like boundaries. It's about time management. It's about administration. It's about having ideas. It's about following through those ideas, about having really shit meetings with people you can't stand … . It's about dealing with homophobia. It's about dealing with other professionals in the health service. (Edward, Midlands)

HIV workers' reliance on an image of professionalism is a phenomenon which has also been pointed out by Cain (1994), albeit within a Canadian context:

> A professional image can help ... workers maintain a sense of competence and expertise in the face of the uncertainty surrounding the epidemic. It is hard to measure the success of their educational efforts, and in the absence of a cure for HIV, their support programs are often experienced as inadequate. By asserting that they are providers of a specialised and professional service, workers claim a status which is more highly valued than that afforded lay practitioners and peer counsellors. This image allows them to interact with doctors and social workers on a more equal footing and helps them successfully compete in an increasingly crowded field of AIDS service providers.
>
> (Cain 1994:52)

Ideas of professionalism were also used by workers to guide their relationships with service users. For example, guidelines about not having sex with clients drew on a notion of professional reputation and a concern not to abuse work relationships. Many spoke about their guidelines in terms of ethics, and saw professional boundaries as part of maintaining a relationship of trust.

Elsewhere, it has been suggested that trust is at the core of professional relationships (Macdonald 1995). In this respect, it is important to consider how the type of work, and relationship to those worked with, is reflected in notions of professionalism. In his book *Mirrors and Masks,* Anslem Strauss (1969) considers the relationship between identification and classification. He argues that:

> An act of classification not only directs overt action but arouses a set of expectations toward the object thus classified.
>
> (Strauss 1969:2)

In relation to people, it clearly matters, therefore, if someone is classified as a volunteer, client or research subject. For example, in a paper on participant observation in saunas, Henriksson and Mansson (1992) describe how they trained gay men to conduct participant observation in Swedish video clubs where sex took place. In many ways their observational role was similar to that of outreach workers. However, in the sauna research, participant observers were allowed to have sex, often using these encounters as material for the research:

> Our rationale for not asking the observers to restrict their participation in sexual encounters is basically not different from the complete observation role that social science textbooks indicate as one of many different observer roles available in observation studies.
>
> (Henriksson and Mansson 1992:4)

It is instructive that having sex whilst working is here legitimised by the desire for reliable data. For outreach workers in this study, more of a counselling and social work[1] legitimisation was brought into play, the intention being to foster more prolonged relationships and provide a service. This highlights the important, if obvious, point that how one's role is defined and legitimised has implications for the way in which boundaries are drawn.

Professionalism also affected perspectives on service provision and the empowerment of service users. Because some gay men may have had bad experiences with other professionals and statutory organisations, some workers said it was particularly important to offer a good service and not abuse their position. For this reason the maintenance of sexual boundaries helped to ensure that men felt able to access the service:

> If I have sex with one of my colleagues from another organisation, who's on a working group that I've set up, then that might not be a good idea because if we then split up ... it gets nasty, then it muddies things ... . But I haven't come between him and services. But, if I'm working with a young man who's just come out, who's very fragile in his gay identity, is having lots of sex, I'm the only person he's spoken to about any of this. I have sex with him, then discard him. Then he's lost a very important route into HIV services and information. (Tim, London)

Professionalism was also brought into play when workers talked of the importance of minimising the influence of personal issues and feelings on work:

> The other thing is that when somebody is rude to you on your outreach work you can't tell them to fuck off. You're a professional person and you're talking to them. (Sanjay, Midlands)

And as Jill put it:

> When someone makes me really mad, you know my professional response would be: 'You know, that's really interesting you say that because you know figures have told us this, that and the other' ... . Whereas if I wasn't being professional, I might say you know: 'Fuck off you dick splash!' (Jill, South)

Like in many other professions, keeping personal interest out of work was seen as key in maintaining integrity and effectiveness. Part of being seen as professional was about maintaining a stance of neutrality and fairness. For example, if workers had sex or made friends with some men it was suggested that this could be seen as favouritism and they would no longer be seen as impartial. Keeping one's personal feelings separate was also seen as important in maintaining a focus on the needs of service users, so as not to cloud workers' judgement:

> As you can imagine, given who some of my ex-boyfriends were ... . They're now working in the field too, and often we have to deal with each other on a

professional level, and it would be unprofessional for me to say: 'Well I don't want to work with your health authority because I hate you', and put the phone down. You know, because you did that to me that one time, whatever. And I wouldn't do it. What I would do is I would try and minimise contact with the person involved. (Jason, London)

Professionalism was thus communicated through boundaries that highlighted the need for equitable service delivery, neutrality and a consistency of approach. There was also a strong emphasis on being non-judgmental and maintaining confidentiality.

Professionalism and sexual identity: an uneasy alliance

Despite the influence that ideas about being professional had on the work and the making of boundaries, several workers felt ambivalent about being seen as a professional. It is important to note that historically it has been 'the professions' that have criminalised and pathologised gay men. For example, it is not so long since homosexuality ceased to be viewed as a mental illness by psychiatrists and doctors. It is perhaps not surprising, therefore, that many gay workers were wary of describing themselves as professionals:

To a certain extent, as a gay man you teach yourself to mistrust authority. You teach yourself to mistrust certainly the NHS, and the police, and your manager, and basically anybody straight … . You basically learn to look after yourself. And to a certain extent there's this bloody great organisation called X NHS Trust which is saying: 'No you're not yourself, you are a very tiny cog in this very large organisation and you will do as you are told' … I mean I am a gay man first and that's what I like to think and I really, I start to dig my heels in if anybody starts to try and undermine that. (Edward, Midlands)

I think professionalism is something that's not been available … to disenfranchised groups on the basis of who they are … . And so I think a lot of people have an aversion to feeling that they are professional, and the service is professional. Because it has all these connotations of elitism, of exclusion, of being an expert, and of being patronising. (Nick, London)

In recent years, this mistrust has at times been compounded by what has come to be described as the de-gaying of AIDS and the professionalisation of the HIV field. As described in Chapter 3, the involvement of professionals in the field, and links with the statutory sector, have been seen by some as having had disastrous consequences for HIV prevention work with gay men. For many gay men there is a clear link between both professionalism and discrimination (McNestry and Hartley 1995), and professionalism and the neglect of gay men's needs, and this can create profound tensions for those workers who, although having strong identities as gay men, also view themselves as professional. There is a tightrope to be walked here that has parallels with wider debates in gay politics about assimilation. As Kinsman (1997) writes:

> In the context of the fight against AIDS, we desperately need state and professional resources and initiatives, and getting them is an important victory. At the same time we have to avoid the implications of state and professional regulatory strategies in limiting and constraining our abilities to organize in our communities and movements.
>
> (Kinsman 1997:233)

For this reason, several writers have commented on the irony of gay men collaborating with medical scientists and government agencies: two areas where, historically, homosexuality has been repressed and oppressed (Plummer 1988; Ryan 1990). This situation is further compounded by the fact that numerous challenges to professionalism and expertise have occurred within the HIV/AIDS field, for example, over the medicalisation of HIV, or the conduct of drug treatment trials (Altman 1994; Campbell 1988; Kinsman 1997; MacLachlan 1992; Treichler 1991).

For a few workers, their sexual and professional identities had become fused. Several described themselves as 'professional gay men':

> It's a sexual job and we're allowed to be a gay man. It's one of the few jobs where you're just allowed to be ... . I went to talk to some probation officers and just sort of, you know, introduced myself as a 'professional poof', and they looked very uncomfortable. They just didn't know whether I was like joking or not. I said: 'Well yeah, I'm paid to be gay, I'm paid because of my experience of getting off with people in clubs ... . Because without those skills, without having hung around clubs for years I wouldn't be able to do the work I'm doing now.' (Andrew, North)

This equating of the job with a certain sexual identity meant that some of the workers felt restrictions on telling those they were not out to as gay men, including relatives, their job titles. On the other hand, they could also feel frustrated that being a professional and being a gay man were seen by others to be incompatible. This was the case both in terms of the perception of other gay men who might mistrust them for 'selling out' and other professionals who, for example, would suggest that gay men are all obsessed with having sex. Workers felt that their gay identity often overrode their identity as a professional, not because they wished it to be this way but because this was how other professionals viewed them. Perhaps, as a result, there was extra pressure put on them to be professional and maintain sexual boundaries:

> When I think about it really early on there was this ... strong current of thinking, particularly in the GU clinic to which I was attached, that I couldn't be a gay man and professional.

K: And why was that, or how was that expressed?

Oh, this intense fear about boundaries. This really kind of fixation on my clothing, um which was just kind of casual and ordinary actually but ...

K: That was seen as unprofessional?

Yeah, yeah. (Tim, London)

I was on an interview panel, and one of the questions was: 'How do you think the notion of boundaries relates to a gay men's HIV prevention officer?' ... . I should have challenged [it]. I wanted to say 'No, it should be how does it relate to health promotion, an HIV prevention officer?' ... . Sometimes I feel there's a subtext that gay men are just very promiscuous basically and need reining in. (Jason, London)

Parkin and Green (1994) have pointed to the sexualisation of gay men in their work on sexuality in residential care settings. They found that gay male care workers' sexuality was frequently seen to be 'problematic, predatory and paedophile'. Consequently, there were pressures on gay male workers to keep their sexuality hidden or to put up with homophobia and sexual innuendo from colleagues. Prejudice from colleagues was also mentioned by some of the men I spoke to and many felt that they were under pressure to represent the gay community in a good light. Other gay workers felt they were subject to criticism for being too personally involved in their work. As Altman (1993) points out, gay men who play a role as community representatives run the risk of both distancing themselves from the gay community and being seen by others as biased if they speak out.

The characteristics of a profession

In Chapter 1, I discussed debates within sociology concerning the definition of professions. I pointed out that although many writers had attempted to identify core defining characteristics of professions, this work has not led to a consensus. However, despite this diversity, there seems to be agreement on certain key characteristics. In an article which looks at professionalism in health and welfare contexts, Williams (1993) cites the following as traits that can be used to characterise professions:

- skill based on theoretical knowledge
- the provision of training and occupation
- tests of the competence of members
- organisation
- adherence to a professional code of conduct
- altruistic service

(Williams, J. 1993:8).

Of course such lists of traits or characteristics are themselves problematic. Johnson (1981) in his book *Professions and Power* criticises trait models for being ahistorical, time bound, atheoretical and limited. Torstendahl (1990) further argues that the differing relationship of the professions to society and the state means that their flexibility is more a defining characteristic than any fixed set of traits. Although trait models may be less than useful for theoretical purposes, they can serve as a useful reflective aid. In the latter part of this chapter I will therefore examine what outreach workers understood by the term 'professional' and compare this with some identified traits.

Professionalism as cultural construct

The emphasis many workers placed on the phrase 'being professional' was striking. Often people would refer to this spontaneously and further probing was necessary to elucidate what was meant. When questioned, workers came up with different answers to this question, though some common themes were identifiable. Many found it hard to give a specific definition:

> God, what is being professional? I mean we use it ourselves. (Toby, North)

> Oh God, I dunno. It's the sort of thing you take for granted isn't it? It's just a word that's used so much, and sort of thrown around without much thought to what it means. (Sarah, London)

Workers' uncertainty seemed to parallel the loose way in which the term was used. As Jason said:

> What does being professional mean? Well I don't know. It's just really difficult isn't it? Some professions have a guide of ethics, have a code of conduct, so it might mean adhering to that. But I'm not involved in a profession like a lawyer, or a doctor, or a teacher, or a counsellor ... . But, being professional is used in a blanket way, and it's used to mean from anything, from meaning you get your mail out really efficiently and quickly, you know: 'very professional', to meaning what we're talking about – sexual boundaries. (Jason, London)

It is interesting to note that here a distinction between 'the professions' (what one person termed 'the white coat sense of the word'), and the more cultural idea of 'being professional' is highlighted. Although undertaking this research has probably sensitised me to the frequent use of the terms such as professional, unprofessional and professionalism, 'being professional' is clearly a construct that is drawn on in a wide range of contexts. For example:

> Marilyn was now freebasing cocaine regularly, which might have explained

his deficient logic. He swore blind that he wasn't basing before he went on stage at Area [a New York club]: 'I would never do that, it's unprofessional.'

(Boy George with Bright 1995:271)

PROFESSIONAL, ATTRACTIVE, slim male, honest and genuine. Seeks similar female for walks, talks, pubs and lunch. Letter, photo. Box 524.

(*Time Out* 1995:159)

[Dr] Margoulies punctuated the thought with an innocent tweak of Bull's clitoris ... From here on in everything that the good doctor did was tantamount to taking a chainsaw to his Tree of Knowledge. For Margoulies had abandoned his professional perspectives, he had allowed his own likes and dislikes to affect his judgment. He was no longer acting in the best interests of his patient.

(Self 1993:127)

Dan Murchie who, sitting to the right of Salter's table suddenly raised his gouty left leg then sounded one of the longest, the loudest, and the most ambitious renditions of bowel music ever to be produced by the anal sphincter. The Fart of the Century, it was a stentorian stinker with the collective energy of a dozen Krakatoas simultaneously blowing their tops. It was a fart with 'professional' written all over it.

(Torrington 1994:155)

It is interesting to note from these examples that the word 'professional' can be used to refer both to identity and to a set of behaviours or practices. So, for example, in the quotes above we can see it being referred to both in terms of rules or ideas about how professionals should behave (not taking drugs, not having sexual contact with patients, not acting in your own interest) and as an identity marker signalling characteristics such as respectability, skill, wealth, career, and being too busy working to find sexual partners. This distinction is important because it illuminates the way in which 'being professional' not only says something about what people do, but also about who they are.

While many workers found defining professional quite difficult, on reflection everyone came up with a definition. Figure 4 on pages 138–9 identifies the main issues mentioned, along with examples of the defining features.

Clearly this list is very different to that produced by Williams. Indeed, comparing the two it would seem that possibly only the last two items from Williams' list (adherence to a professional code of conduct and altruistic service) appear in the items listed in Figure 4. For example, in the table no attention is paid to things such as access to specialised knowledge that is often seen as defining the professions. Instead, there is a focus on the mechanics of actually carrying out work, and references to the organisational settings in which work takes place. Significantly, the list generated by outreach workers also emphasises the emotion work involved in being a professional.

Comparing the list in Figure 4 with Williams' criteria is illuminating in that it highlights some of the tensions workers experienced between traditional notions of what being professional meant, and how they personally wanted to work, or what they valued. In order to explore these issues the remainder of this chapter is divided into sections addressing some of the differing definitions of being professional outlined. This discussion identifies the reasons why professionalism and sexual identity sometimes have a problematic relationship in HIV-related work.

'Walk it like you talk it': experience, expertise and knowledge

The professions have been defined as knowledge-based occupations (Larson 1977, 1990; Torstendahl 1990). Although sociologically, many health services are often described as semi-professions, and thus not seen as true professions, it is perhaps useful to reflect on the idea of HIV prevention as a knowledge-based occupation to see what this reveals about the term 'professional' and the apparent contradictions it may cause. One of the immediate questions raised is the difference between taught knowledge and life experience. The former is classically taken to be a defining feature of the professions, and the latter was frequently mentioned as the primary qualification for those doing HIV prevention work with gay men. But is there a difference between knowledge and experience? The *Collins English Dictionary* defines the primary meaning of 'experienced' as:

> Having become skilful or knowledgeable from extensive contact or participation or observation.
>
> (*Collins English Dictionary* 1990:536)

and defines experience as meaning:

> direct personal participation or observation; actual knowledge, or contact … accumulated knowledge esp of practical matters.
>
> (*Collins English Dictionary* 1990:536)

This definition is suggestive both of a link between experience and knowledge, and the variety of ways in which knowledge can be gained through experience. It emphasises both contact and participation, the major qualifications that many men suggested they brought to the work through their life experience as gay or bisexual men.[2]

Consider next, a dictionary definition of knowledge:

> knowledge – the facts, feelings or experiences known by a person or a group of people … awareness, consciousness or familiarity gained by experience or learning … informed learning, specific information about a subject.
>
> (*Collins English Dictionary* 1990:849)

Definitions generated from interviews	Examples given in interviews
Focusing on a task	Having a clear plan about what you are doing, why and with whom; clear aim; knowing what the work involves and what you need to do; setting objectives; developing policies
Providing a service	Providing a service well, delivering a contract, quality and effectiveness; ensuring that resources are used effectively; doing the best you can; giving best advice; confident in your information; eliciting information without upsetting people; getting mail out quickly; finding out information you don't know; being aware of how you're working
Equitable service delivery	Being non-judgmental; contacting a wide variety of people
Boundaries	Not displaying inappropriate behaviour, e.g. drinking alcohol, taking drugs; adherence to a code of conduct; not having sex with clients; not expecting needs for sex and intimacy to be met through work; a private life that doesn't denigrate work; confidentiality; learning when to say no; knowing your limits
Living the job	Identity; vocation; a permanent work related role
Being responsible	Being responsible to communities and users; explaining your actions to people; instilling confidence in others
Credible to a wide range of people	Tailoring work; adapting to different people and environments; using appropriate language, dressing appropriately
Detachment	Controlling feelings; being appropriately emotional; not reacting personally; not bringing personal issues into work; not being rude to people; not hugging or kissing people as a greeting at work; not losing temper; keeping distance and not being 'one of the lads'; maintaining neutrality; avoiding 'bitchy' comments when socialising
Being paid	Responsible to funders
Aware of relationship to wider system	Line management and filling in forms; public role; using supervision

Access to privileged information	Power to use information; using information to help others
Authoritative role	Authority; being competent; having a smart title; understanding theory behind the work; upholding what the project stands for; being a role model
Being ethical	Respecting confidentiality
Responding to needs	Promoting the needs of communities worked with and empowering them.

Figure 4 Definitions of the term 'professional'.

Here, learning, training and theoretical knowledge are emphasised. In fact, it is the possession of an expert, systematised and theoretical body of knowledge that is seen as vital for any occupation wishing to professionalise. As Macdonald writes:

> The lay person has no means of knowing objectively whether the professional can in fact provide the service on offer, and must therefore make a judgement on other criteria. In fact the professional has to be taken on trust and so is keen to display those characteristics which are believed to represent trustworthiness. These will include evidence of training and knowledge acquired – degrees, diplomas and certificates.
>
> (Macdonald 1992:3)

As we have already seen, because of historical (and in some cases continued) negative responses by professions, such characteristics are not necessarily going to be seen as evidence of trust by gay and bisexual men (see King 1995).

It is perhaps not surprising that workers themselves saw sexual identity as crucially important to professionalism; as one worker said: 'being gay is our expertise'. This is quite different from the usual idea of expertise gained through professional training and formal qualifications (Crompton and Sanderson 1990). Among outreach workers, the view most usually expressed was that life experience and insights gained from having a gay sexual identity were the most useful qualifying characteristics. This view recognised the importance of community-based work and the need for culturally appropriate and rooted HIV prevention initiatives (Daly and Horton 1993).

A small number of the male workers felt that the idea of their sexuality *per se* as the qualification for their employment generated difficulties. For example, an over emphasis on the link between life experience and identity resulted in knowledge and experience being seen as an automatic consequence of sexual identity. As not all gay men have had the same life experiences, some workers felt that appeals to shared experience led to a neglect of the variety and diversity of gay and bisexual men's experiences (see also Altman 1993; Prout and Deverell 1995; Sandfort 1995). For example, it was suggested that the re-gaying of AIDS in the mid-1990s had led to something of a 'Sohoisation' of AIDS whereby certain gay men's needs and desires[3] had assumed to be those of all gay men. In addition, the re-gaying of the epidemic was seen to have encouraged reductionist arguments about who is actually qualified to do the work. The result of this was that women, who have historically been involved in HIV prevention with gay and bisexual men in the UK, felt that they were no longer seen to have valid skills and knowledge to offer.

The idea of there being an automatic link between knowledge and identity was also seen to mask the fact that gay man too had gone through a process of learning. Some talked about how, before their employment, they had not had personal experience of certain activities such as anal sex, cruising, or public sex environments, even though they were assumed to have had them. Although much was made of the fact that women would be limited in the work because of their gender and sexuality, the constraining effects of other sexualities were more rarely discussed. In fact, for all the emphasis on the importance of sexuality and sexual skills, a quarter of those interviewed said that there had been times when (potential) service users had not even realised they were gay. Although most people felt that having a gay or bisexual identity, or at least having sex with men, was an important experience to bring to the job, many pointed out that there was a need to emphasise the other skills and qualities needed for outreach work, and for these to be validated. Not all gay men make good outreach workers, and there is a need to understand that knowledge and expertise can be gained in different ways.

The late 1990s saw an increase in the amount and type of training available to those working with gay men, coupled with more gay men's workers holding health promotion qualifications. It will be interesting to see whether the growing body of experience in relation to gay and bisexual men's HIV prevention will become more formalised as the field professionalises.

Being a client and a professional: non-distanced relationships

There is an obvious difference in the workers' roles to those of many other professionals. Outreach workers are not paid directly by clients for providing a service. Moreover, they offer their services freely, rather than waiting to be approached:

> I think when you are doing outreach on the scene and things like that people … see you as one of them. If you are doing it in an office, if somebody comes to you in an office, you are a professional worker, do you know what I mean? It's that difference. And the power structure seems different, the power

relationship feels different. It seems you're on a more of an equal level if you are out in a club. (Sean, North)

Despite an interest in appearing professional, constructs of 'professionalism' were questioned by many for, as gay men themselves, workers were part of the client group, and several had an emotional and political motivation for doing the work:

> The reason why I got into this job was because I had a keen interest in seeing HIV prevention done amongst gay men … . And because politically I wanted to be involved in a job that had something to say to me personally, something that gave me some kind of personal fulfilment, and about which I knew a lot. Because I've been involved in like, gay politics and gay organisations for a long time. (Sean, North)

At times, workers' sense of being professional was less strong than other identities related to, for example, sexuality or ethnicity. This meant that relationships with service users were very different from those considered to be the norm for other professionals:

> I think the nature of the work concerned, it's like, because you're working with men who have sex with men, and you are yourself a man who has sex with men and so on, a lot of the issues … are issues that concern you as well not just because you're working … . Particularly as a black worker working in a Black project for men who have sex with men. It's like this, you know minority within a minority really. You do feel this duty really to do the work… . It's almost like if you weren't being paid you'd feel this duty to do it, because it's about helping your own people. (Isaac, Midlands)

On the whole, workers were less interested in increasing the distance between themselves and service users or clients than in working on the basis of a shared sexual identity or at least the shared experience of having sex with men. As part of the client group, workers were in fact potential consumers as well as providers of services, an issue rarely considered in the sociological literature on professions. Rather than using constructs of professionalism as a way of asserting power and distance over fee-paying clients, gay and bisexual workers used these notions to assert their expertise as gay men within organisations. Their experiences suggest that it is important to consider professionalism not just as a means of regulating the relationship between the provider of a service and the consumer, but also as a way of behaving and as an identity.

In the last twenty years various social and political movements have led to the emergence of what has been called a 'new public health'. This has been codified in the Ottawa Charter for Health promotion (1986) (a declaration adopted by thirty-eight countries), and other health promotion policy initiatives that have emphasised, amongst other things, the need for a style of work that is needs led and owned by communities (Ashton and Seymour 1988). There has been a move towards recognising the skills and experiences of service users in determining their own health needs and behaviours, together with a style of health promotion which encourages professionals to work in partnership with communities. Such ideas of partnership can be seen as challenging the traditional expert and pedagogical role of the health professional who becomes an involved guide and advocate rather than a distant educator and expert (Williams, J. 1993). This emphasis on involvement and partnership is also expressed by holistic health workers (Deverell and Sharma 2000). In this way, outreach workers' challenges to ideas of professionalism can be seen as part of a wider move to change the nature of working relationships in health-related fields.

The personal is professional

One aspect of professionalism that was felt to be important by the majority of those interviewed was not bringing personal issues into the work. Elsewhere, this form of behaviour has often been associated with the idea of being professional. For example, in the novel *The Remains of the Day*, Stevens, the butler, discusses what distinguishes a great butler from a merely competent one. It is, he argues, a matter of dignity:

> 'Dignity' has to do crucially with a butler's ability not to abandon the professional being he inhabits. Lesser butlers will abandon their professional being for the private one at the least provocation. For such persons, being a butler is like playing some pantomime role; a small push, a slight stumble, and the facade will drop off to reveal the actor underneath. The great butlers are great by virtue of their ability to inhabit their professional role and inhabit it to the utmost; they will not be shaken out by external events, however surprising, alarming or vexing.
>
> (Ishiguro 1990:42–3)

Comparable ideas about professionalism had clearly been internalised by some of the workers, who strove to keep their personal views and feelings out of their work. This involved trying to remain non-judgmental, providing an equitable service to all those worked with, not shouting in meetings, concentrating on the needs of those worked with, and not displaying sexual arousal. But workers also identified a more vocational aspect to their employment. As Toby put it:

> This work relies on being more than professional … it's got to do with what I was saying about vocation, and I think you've got to do it with vigour and with enthusiasm and with passion … I suppose I see being professional as being a basic set of core, like ethical, being ethical if you like. But I don't think this work will succeed if you're just that. (Toby, North)

Many emphasised the importance of having community connections and were concerned that having too professional an image might distance them from the men with whom they worked. Being part of the local community, and being seen to have had similar experiences and difficulties, was the way in which to build trust. This led some to suggest that there was a need for a new definition of professionalism, one that recognised the usefulness of shared experience. As Erkan explained:

> It's about other people appreciating where the normal, or what's conceived to be the accepted boundaries, are sometimes not always the accepted boundaries between gay workers and gay clients … . It's where the clients will need you to relate to them in a framework other than the straight world. Or where, for example, the subtext of where you both socialise comes in, or the slang words you might both use … . Or the kind of similar oppression that you're both subjected to, similar discriminations that you've both had, where you're just going to have to acknowledge that within the counselling relationship, or within the professional relationship … . It has a different texture to it … . The boundaries need to be kept in check of really tightly. But I think gay workers, that I've seen, good gay workers have been able to judge when and where to relax them, just so far without confusing the clients. (Erkan, London)

Although at times valuable, being close to those worked with could prove difficult. People could feel permanently at work or might experience similar anxieties to those they were supporting:

> I used to think that I could work with HIV issues quite, in a detached sense … . It was like so far away from me that, I'd be able to work in a really professional way with it. I've kind of got a lot more involved with my own personal issues … really worried about my own (HIV) status and testing issues and all that kind of thing. And maybe now I feel that I'm at my most ineffective in relation to HIV work. (Erkan, London)

> When issues come up in your personal life, your professional ability to do your job is brought into question. The fact that you still have issues [around safer sex] makes you feel that when you have been talking to people professionally, you haven't really been engaging with what it must be like. (Peter, East)

Interestingly, there are moves in occupations such as health promotion, social work and nursing towards a new understanding of professionalism which gives greater recognition to the importance of the 'self' or personal qualities of the professional; most particularly their interpersonal skills and intuition (Williams, J. 1993). As Johnson has argued:

> affective neutrality and professional authority – the latter stemming from

professional competence – are likely to operate only where they do not conflict with other and more important aspects of the relationship between professional and client.

(Johnson 1981:36)

That said, the development of these understandings, in which the personal is seen as a potential resource to be drawn upon, sits uncomfortably with more conventional definitions of professionalism. It also means that workers can need greater emotional support.

One of us, one of them, or one of those: payment and professionalisation

Three of the eight definitions of professional in the *Collins English Dictionary* (1990) make explicit reference to payment. The fact that at the level of cultural understanding, being professional means being paid, highlights a major tension for many gay men in HIV work. For those whose primary motivation for doing the work is linked to a political and altruistic desire to prevent others becoming infected, labelling themselves as professional is something of a contradiction. Although most workers enjoyed having a salary, most actively resisted seeing payment as their reason for doing the work. Their unease was clearly related to wider debates within HIV work about professionalism and in particular the increasing professionalisation of AIDS voluntary organisations (Weeks *et al.* 1994). For example, there has long been cynicism about people who are 'AIDS professionals' rather than being personally committed to the work (MacLachlan 1992). Sometimes this has extended to a distrust of heterosexuals, or even to those who are (or were assumed to be) HIV negative (see Kennett 1995):

> I had some really bad experiences when I first got involved in this work ... and I was made to feel very, very guilty ... . 'Well you don't know how lucky you are' and you know ... 'What can you possibly know, you can't possibly know what it's like to live with this virus' ... . And that was very hard to work that one through, because it's about ... it's like, you know, legitimising your existence. (Keith, North)

The value placed on personal experience could also be seen in the way in which credibility in the HIV field at the time of the fieldwork sometimes appeared to relate to the number of people you knew who had died from HIV disease. Assumed links between sexual identity and personal experience of HIV meant that assumptions tended to be made about who had been personally affected and who had not (see also Maslanka 1993). As Jill said:[4]

> Straight people and women have their grief around HIV as well, but that's not assumed about you I think ... . There's more often the assumption that you're doing it because it's a good job, or you're CV collecting or whatever,

rather than personal commitment you know. I think there's a lot of that. (Jill, South)

In part, this situation may have its origins in the historic links between HIV prevention, volunteerism and gay activism. Among outreach workers the term 'professional' was used to refer not just to those who are paid, but also to those who are not truly committed to the cause and simply interested in their careers. Several people mentioned that within the HIV field a common way of disparaging someone's work or questioning their commitment has been to label them as being 'too professional'[5]. As one worker commented, 'Professional is a hurtful word'. It is perhaps therefore not surprising that some people did not feel happy embracing it.

Some of these issues came to the fore in arguments about the re-gaying of AIDS. For example, in an article describing sexual boundaries as unnecessarily professional and bureaucratic, King (1993b) argues that boundaries themselves are a manifestation of the de-gaying and professionalisation of AIDS organisations, where gay identity has become secondary to professional identity:

> In the mid-1980s, when safer sex campaigns led to unprecedented behaviour changes among gay men, understanding and spreading the word about safer sex was something that any gay man could do in his everyday life. But in the De-gaying Years, AIDS education came to be seen as a job for professional employees. In the unusual event of any HIV-prevention campaigns being targeted at gay men, safer sex education became something done to gay men by nine-to-five experts working to codes of conduct.
>
> (King 1993b:14)

King (1993b) further argued that: 'Boundaries actively obstruct effective forms of outreach work' by preventing workers from passing safer sex messages by having safer sex. This criticism was initially taken up by British organisations such as Gay Men Fighting AIDS (GMFA), which was set up to do prevention work specifically for gay men[6] (see Chapter 3):

> GMFA has caused a bit of a stir with our very personal way of promoting safer sex. Unlike some other organisations, we don't forbid our volunteers from having sex with 'clients'. Indeed we see it as the essential way gay men can promote safer sex. We don't see ourselves as separate from other gay men, rather we see [ourselves] as part of a community and as part of a safer sex movement within that community.

> This seems to have rattled some outsiders who are confused by our 'professional boundaries'. The implication is that our priorities and responsibilities are unclear. While they may be unclear to people outside GMFA, they seem clear enough to our volunteers. We agree to put the project first ... we

don't spend the whole time in bushes demonstrating blowjobs. We save that for tea breaks.

(Dockrell 1993:1)

This emphasis on direct community involvement upset some other gay men's workers who also felt very much part of the community but did not have the same freedom as GMFA volunteers. For example, as health authority employees, many were subject to codes of conduct. All the workers interviewed were also concerned to avoid doing anything that might bring their project into disrepute and thus affect the continuity of the work. This was particularly the case because, having fought hard for funding, they did not want to endanger the work by having sex with men who could be construed as clients. As one health authority worker said in response to the above criticism:

> I mean, they've set up this thing about, you know, the normal boring HIV professionals who don't agree with that model, and we who know. When actually the normal boring HIV prevention workers know that they want people to tell their lovers, and of course want people to have sex. But what they [also] know is that for paid workers in that formal set up to do that … is not necessarily ethical, and is generally not practical. (Jason, London)

Contemporary articles about outreach and boundaries written from a re-gaying perspective were mentioned by several workers who felt unfairly criticised, and upset that their identity as gay men was being overlooked, because they were paid or worked in the statutory sector, or both. The fact that Peter Scott, a major figure in the UK re-gaying movement, described those gay male workers employed in the statutory sector as: 'a collaborating class of gay men, ineffectual or outnumbered' (in Garfield 1994:130), not surprisingly made many feel insulted. This was particularly so for those who felt they had often worked hard and made major gains locally by promoting the needs of gay men. As paid workers, they did not have the same freedoms as GMFA volunteers, but they wanted their experience and commitment as gay men to be recognised. As Bill (Midlands) said in relation to a newspaper article:

> I found his [King's] criticisms about [boundaries], I think one reference he used, or a sentence he used was you know sort of 'Lo and behold, and they can never have sex with the men that they're serving'. I found that extremely annoying because I wouldn't sacrifice myself for my work. I would not do that. And the situation just does not exist for me to be able to do that. And to criticise me for not doing that then I. I took it as a personal affront and that's the way I see it. Because there are, as I said earlier, constraints around what I can and can't do. (Bill, Midlands)

Workers also expressed reservations about GMFA's claim that having safer sex with service users was an effective form of peer education:[7]

You know, when people are talking about … um … well it might be peer education to have sex with the people you are working with, I just think that's silly … . If you want to have a shag with the people you're working with, and you don't care about boundaries, then just say that really. To make out that it's *peer education*, I just think is undignified really. I mean where's your quality control if it's peer education *(laughs)*? Where's your equal opportunities? Where's your evaluation? … What if the person, you know, employed, well volunteering, for your organisation has unprotected sex, as indeed they might … . Then what kind of peer education is that? (Tim, London)

Workers sometimes expressed frustration at the division that had been set up between professionals and gay men because they felt they were both. Indeed, some pointed out that they demonstrated their commitment to not becoming an 'overriding professional' by maintaining their capacity to relate personally to service users:

Being too professional is … . There's two workers I know quite well, *(laughs)* who will not allow any physical contact with them, from the rentboys for example. Um … you know whether that's a peck on the cheek, a hand on the knee while they're sat talking in Burger King, sometimes a cuddle … . What I often see is that clients start rejecting 'em … they start treating 'em on this superficial: 'Oh you're the worker, I will only tell you what you need to know, and what you ask me'. On the other side of that, is the worker who wears inappropriate clothing that invites unwarranted [physical] advances … . So it goes the other way. But for me, it's [professional] about being in the middle, being flexible. (Derek, London)

Part of the criticism that has developed around boundaries arises from a view of HIV prevention as a peer activity, rather than a health promotion service. Much HIV prevention is now undertaken by those who are paid and the distinction between commitment and career seems inadequate. However, the strength of feeling that the word 'professional' can arouse highlights the need to recognise the role that personal commitment, community involvement and politics continue to play in the work.

'It's the condom man': the merging of professional and sexual identity

A final issue of importance concerning the relationship between sexual identity and professionalism is the vocational aspect of the work, or the identity element of being professional. In the 1990s, the number of gay and bisexual men's workers carrying out outreach work on the gay scene led some to suggest that HIV prevention workers had become visible and identifiable characters. For example:

I can usually spot one a mile off. It's something to do with his haircut, the style of his clothes, and the ubiquitous shoulder bag which seems to accompany him everywhere.

(Harrison 1994:55)

If you ain't got a shaved head, big boots and a muscular bum, you ain't nobody. A friend of mine was complaining about the days of preparation and careful thought needed to be considered for a job in gay men's outreach recently. 'Filling in the job application form?' I asked sympathetically. 'No', he replied, 'butching up for the interview'.

(Power 1993:269)

Several of those interviewed also joked about the developing image of the HIV outreach worker. Some talked about becoming marked out from the rest of the gay community.[8] This was particularly the case for those working in smaller towns. As one worker put it:

You're always known for your work rather than say, for example, the size of your dick, *(laughs)* which is what most other men on the scene are known about. (Edward, Midlands)

When socialising on their local gay scene outside work, many reported that they tended to be seen as a worker rather than just another gay man, and so potential sexual partners would often not approach them. A few interviewees also found it hard to encourage contact with some men during work sessions as these men feared identifying themselves as HIV positive, or as having a concern, if their friends saw them talking to a worker. This raises interesting issues for community based ways of working that emphasise the importance of being part of the community, or being seen as a peer.

In larger towns, the situation was slightly different. Here, some workers described how they had started to socialise mainly with other gay men involved in HIV prevention. This led some to feel separated from the experiences and needs of other gay men. As Tim explained:

You become part of a community of workers, and a kind of culture of HIV work, and become kind of socialised into that. Where it's very easy to talk about sex, comparatively very easy to be gay … very. Well, maybe not easy to have an HIV test, that's ridiculous. But it's part of your social currency that people may have HIV tests you know, and have comparatively good support around, around sexual health. And that's a boundary that also needs addressing. (Tim, London)

Most of the workers interviewed had strong identities both as gay men and as professionals, although which of these was most dominant at any time varied. Some felt torn between their different identities and the different communities to which they belonged. For George, professional identity was seen to be the most prominent when he was working:

> My line is that if I'm working on the streets, in a sense my sexuality is secondary to being a worker. And though I use my sexuality, I'm there as a worker, not necessarily as a gay man. Though I don't think I could do this work unless I was a gay man. I know that with that pay packet and with that contract comes a responsibility. (George, North)

However, context was crucial in determining role, for in a meeting with other professionals who were being heterosexist, or when putting forward the needs of gay men, this same worker felt that his gay identity became more important. Another worker, Edward, who liked to think he was a gay man first, and professional second, was aware that at times his identity as a worker led him to behave in certain ways:

> I know that I can't just go to a users, a user or a purchaser meeting in the middle of town and say: 'I am a gay man in [this town] and I think this service should be changed to that' ... I've got to remember that to a certain extent [that here] I am a professional first, and there are certain things I can say and certain things I can't say. (Edward, Midlands)

In fact, for most men interviewed both identities were interlinked and difficult to separate.

Conclusions

This chapter has explored some of the issues that arose for gay men's workers in relation to being 'professional'. Although not seeing themselves as a profession, workers clearly drew on cultural notions of what being professional meant and emphasised the importance of being seen to 'be professional' in their dealings with funders, clients and the wider community. To some extent, this was linked to the broader culture of the UK health service and the need for a respectable and organised image in order successfully to compete for funding. Being 'professional' was also seen as a good defence against attacks from the tabloid press or others.

However, many workers felt ambivalent about calling themselves professionals, and some actively resisted it. The historical development of HIV prevention, discrimination against gay men by the professions, the importance of community based ways of working, and a desire not to be detached and distanced were all factors at work. These contradictions and anxieties made it very difficult for those workers with strong identities as gay men who also wanted to be professional. Retaining credibility, both among other professionals and other gay and bisexual men, while maintaining a sense of integrity and political commitment, could be very stressful.

Developing roles in a new occupational field, workers were to some extent caught up in a process of defining appropriate professional conduct. Trying to do this around a set of political commitments that have consistently challenged professional groups and notions of professionalism proved difficult. This was particularly the case given that the term 'professional' has been used disparagingly in HIV work: being used to criticise people for a multitude of 'sins' such as being heterosexual, being paid, having qualifications or working in the statutory sector. Although these factors may be related, and at times overlap, they are significantly different. It is therefore unfortunate that important arguments concerning the neglect of gay men's needs, and the value of community based work with gay and bisexual men, have at times been confused with a rejection of professionalism. Certainly, for workers, being professional could be important in developing new services and carrying out work successfully. Indeed, some saw appeals to professionalism as a way of improving services for gay and bisexual men, and ensuring that the needs of gay and bisexual men were more widely recognised.

8   Professionalism and
work–life balance

An examination of outreach workers' experiences raises important issues not just for HIV prevention but also for a wide range of occupations. In this final chapter, I will discuss key findings and their implications through a focus on three themes: professionalism; emotion work; and boundaries of home, sex and work. Through a discussion of new ideas about professionalism and the work–life balance the applicability of the issues raised in this study to contemporary debates about work and professionalism is explored.

Professionalism

> The professional discourse has a momentum of its own … . The structures developed become the criteria and standards of proper professional performance. Being a professional involves knowing how to do it this way, how to produce work that conforms to these standards, addressing these topics, and following these methodologies. Further, doing it this way is how we recognise ourselves as professionals.
>
> (Smith 1988:60)

Organisational ideals about the purpose and performance of work are expressed through understandings of professionalism and the management of various types of boundary. Through learning the standards and expectations required in a job workers are socialised into professional behaviour. Hochschild has discussed this in her work on flight attendants:

> Like workers in many other occupations, they call themselves 'professional' because they have mastered a body of knowledge and want respect for that. Companies also use 'professional' to refer to this knowledge, but they refer to something else as well. For them a 'professional' flight attendant is one who has completely accepted the rules of standardization. The flight attendant who most nearly meets the appearance code ideal is therefore 'the most professional' in this regard.
>
> (Hochschild 1983:103)

In this way, organisational codes of conduct and ideas of 'appropriate' behaviour link individual workers to organisational values. In more established occupations this is usually achieved through standardised processes of training and socialisation and agreed codes of conduct. However, in every job there is always an element of learning what behaviours are required for the role:

> What a job description rarely does is to set out the expectations which we can legitimately have of others with whom we will be working, such as colleagues, superiors and other professionals, as well as users and their families. While it may be clear what our duties are, we have to discover what kinds of relationship are possible and desirable, as well as required, in the new situation.
>
> Lyon 1993:237)

This study showed that organisations often did not have clear ideas themselves about what being a professional outreach worker meant. In the early 1990s in the UK, formal training and established codes of conduct were rare. As Tim said, describing why he had developed a boundary-related training course for gay men's workers:

> We were very aware that very few people actually addressed that stuff with gay men really, that they're just kind of put in post and expected to have the boundaries really. You know whereas if you go on a social work course, you know, a lot of it is implicitly or explicitly about where your boundaries are. (Tim, London)

In interviews, outreach workers stressed the importance of training, management support and supervision both in helping them to legitimise boundary issues as part of work, and in helping to make boundary management part of an organisational process. However, developing an agreed set of boundaries between workers and managers was not necessarily a straightforward process, and often involved a great deal of negotiation. Developing understandings of appropriate behaviour frequently involved workers challenging and resisting the ideas that managers or organisations put forward. Outreach workers' experiences highlight the fact that although the rhetoric of professionalism can bring workers into line with organisational aims, learning to be professional is a much more active process than just internalising norms and values.

Outreach workers' ideas about appropriate behaviour were learned through experience:

> So many workers come into this field without formal training. I mean … unfortunately they don't do degrees in gay men's outreach work, and nobody really knows what they're doing to start with. (Edward, Midlands)

Over time, workers developed a stronger sense of what was required and began to internalise ideas about professionalism and boundary making in order to manage their own behaviour. As outlined in Chapter 4, workers talked of developing a work mentality or focus in order to guide their behaviour both within work and outside of it. Foucault (1979) has argued that this kind of self-regulation has become the most common form of modern day bureaucratic control, replacing more overt management control and sanctions. Certainly, Hearn and Parkin suggest that for those involved in 'people work' organisational control exists through the management of emotions, 'professionalism', 'institutional agencies' and a reliance on informal group support (1987:89). This kind of self-management was reflected in outreach workers' continual reference to the need to be 'professional' and their criticism of others for being either too professional, or not professional enough. In this way, ideals of professionalism were used to signify appropriate standards and expectations and served as a form of peer control.

Knowledge and expertise

> The origins of any profession lie in the existence of an area of knowledge which those who possess it are able to isolate from social knowledge generally, and establish a special claim to. As important as retaining control of it, is its development and presentation to society as the special province of the members, who alone can be trusted to use it in an ethical manner.
>
> (Macdonald 1995:xiii)

Specialised knowledge has been seen as a key characteristic of the professions in much sociological work. Indeed, Macdonald (1995) argues that it has been the emphasis on the importance of practice, rather than knowledge, in the caring professions that has devalued these occupations and made it harder for them to achieve professional status. Certainly, knowledge as the foundation for claims to professionalism within health promotion can be challenged. As Williams has pointed out, much health promotion knowledge should in fact be regarded as the 'best available opinion', given that so little of it has been subject to rigorous testing (Williams, J. 1993:11). Where the means of helping people is through the personal relationship, the effectiveness of the working relationship depends more on the quality of the relationship between clients and professionals than on the use of expert knowledge:

> Professional practice from this perspective has less to do with the application of esoteric knowledge, more to do with intuition, common sense, techniques for helping and interpersonal skills … . The primary focus of professional training thus becomes, not the inculcation of a body of expert knowledge, but the identification and development of personal and interpersonal skills; and professional knowledge has a lower priority than the quality of the professional's relationship with the client.
>
> (Williams, J. 1993:13)

Elsewhere, Rueschmeyer (1983) suggests that knowledge may play a more limited role in professional relationships than has previously been assumed. Indeed, Davies (1996) has argued that the new managerialism and feminism have changed ideas about professional behaviour. This can be seen in the development of a new model for professional practice, which moves away from expert and theoretical knowledge to emphasise interpersonal skills. Importantly, only one interviewee in this study spoke about professionalism in terms of knowledge. Instead outreach workers' everyday understandings of professionalism referred much more to identity and practices. It was this emphasis on ways of being and doing that led several interviewees to suggest that different definitions of what it meant to be professional needed to be adopted. For example, it was possible to be 'professional' whilst being naked, wearing jeans or drinking a pint of beer. The analysis of workers' own understandings of professionalism highlighted the need to consider professionalism not just as a process of social closure, but to think of it as a discourse which shapes relationships to the self, organisations and service users.

Trust and respect

Macdonald (1995) has noted that trust is fundamental to the professional relationship, and the stress on respectability is an important way in which 'the professions' encourage others to place trust in them. Williams (1993) argues that in order to enhance status and signal trust, more occupations are trying to professionalise. This is particularly the case in the increasingly competitive environment in which both voluntary organisations and the health service compete for funds:

> the 'operating environment' for voluntary organisations has become more highly regulated, more competitive and more output-driven. In this context ... potential conflicts arise between the aim of 'doing good' in relation to social issues and causes, and the pressures of 'doing well' as organisations in an increasingly professional and competitive environment.
>
> (Tonkiss and Passey 1999:261)

The stress outreach workers and their managers placed on 'being professional' was clearly linked to this need to be seen to be providing a valued service. One of the main reasons why respectability and credibility were so important to outreach workers was that they had to communicate to others the skills and expertise needed for the work. The close links of the work with HIV and gay men meant that they often feared public exposure, and suffered hostile reactions from some quarters – including at times their own organisations:

> To a certain extent we're under a bit of a contradiction in the fact that they [NHS Trust] want us to have a high profile service, and yet they don't want it to be so high profile that like people like [the local newspaper] will get hold of it. (Edward, Midlands)

The sexual nature of the work also meant that it was easily discredited. This in turn meant that any process of professionalisation was not straightforward. For outreach workers such as those interviewed here, carving out a specialised role involved convincing others that they had relevant expertise and that the services they could provide were important to HIV prevention. In this respect, outreach workers had to work hard to establish the legitimacy of their practice (Macdonald 1995).

In recent years, and as HIV prevention work has become more integrated into broader sexual health programmes, the work itself has become more established and accepted. Outreach work with gay men that was once seen as risky and radical is now more acceptable both as an occupation and as a method of HIV prevention. Indeed, as the amount of funded HIV prevention work itself decreases, those who remain working in this area seem to be finding ways to reconcile their personal and political desires to improve the lives of gay men with the taking on of a more professional health role. This can be seen in the greater use of health promotion and psychology theories, an emphasis on research and evaluation, a growth in the number of workers studying for health related qualifications and the merger of voluntary organisations which previously held distinct political views.

Professionalism and identity

Within sociology, it is now commonplace to assert that people have more than one identity; as Weeks writes:

> Identity is about belonging, about what you have in common with some people and what differentiates you from others. At its most basic it gives you a sense of personal location, the stable core to your individuality. But it is also about your social relationships, your complex involvement with others, and in the modern world these have become ever more complex and confusing. Each of us live with a variety of potentially contradictory identities, which battle within us for allegiance.
>
> (Weeks 1990:88)

This raises interesting questions about the balancing of professional and other identities within work. O'Brien (1994) writes that, historically, nurses have placed importance on being the right sort of person to do the work, rather than having technical competence, emphasising life experience and personal qualities above training and knowledge. Furthermore, he argues that the nurses he interviewed saw their skills in forming and working with relationships as derived mainly from their experience as women:

> The formation of a specific type of relationship appears as a necessary component of their health provider roles. At the same time, the skills they possessed in fulfilling the relationship-forming task were argued to derive, not from the

qualities of being a *nurse* but from the qualities of being a *woman*. That is, they perceived a direct overlap between their 'public' functions and 'private' identities.

(O'Brien 1994:399)

There are clear parallels here with the emphasis male outreach workers placed on their skills as gay or bisexual men as the primary qualification for undertaking outreach. Their desire to minimise the social distance between themselves and clients through membership of a shared community involved emphasising different kinds of experience:

> One of the qualifications that I have for this job is the fact that I'm a young gay man ... . My life experience is qualification in itself, and my anger, and my emotional response are qualifications ... [It's] actually recognising human elements, rather than just sort of like working within a framework of like ... academia. (Keith, North)

This focus on gay expertise could be seen as a bargaining tool which workers used to maintain control over their work and safeguard their occupational role. However, it also reflects the historical situation, outlined in Chapter 3, in which HIV prevention developed from community based initiatives rather than originating in more mainstream forms of health promotion. The fact that most workers had been employed because of their links to the gay community also downplayed the importance of health-related qualifications. This highlights an important difference to the nurses O'Brien mentions. Although nurses may emphasise and use 'womanly' qualities, the need for these characteristics is not advertised in as explicit a way as those in outreach workers' job descriptions. Indeed, while all professionals will share some personal characteristics with their clients, this is rarely seen as the basis for the working relationship.

In his work on gay and lesbian police officers, Marc Burke has highlighted the tension that can be experienced between professional and sexual identities:

> If the policeman's lot 'is not a happy one', then the plight of the gay or lesbian police officer is far worse. To begin with, although homosexuality is not proscribed in the police by legislation as it is in the armed forces that has not made it any more professionally acceptable. The resultant exploitable combination of 'police officer' and 'homosexual' has resulted in a tradition of considering such persons as unsuited for police work by virtue of their security threat ... . Secondly, where homosexual officers opt to declare their orientation, they court stigmatization in both of their major life roles: As police officers they may be rejected by the community at large and particularly by some sections of the lesbian and gay communities as '(fascist) pigs', whilst in their lives at work they may be ridiculed and discriminated against by their colleagues as 'poofs' or 'lezzies'.

(Burke 1994:3)

His work examines the extent to which officers live 'double' as opposed to 'integrated' lives, and whether their police or sexual identities are dominant. He develops a four stage 'gay police career' model to show how individuals progress through a process whereby a rounded and 'integrated' sense of self emerges only after their 'police' and 'gay' identities have been successfully reconciled. Burke points out that 'identity dominance is a manifestation of an officer's orientational and occupational development at a given period of time'; I would suggest that an exploration of these periods of time, or contexts may be more useful. Certainly, among outreach workers the question of which identity was strongest depended on where they were, who they were with, their personal politics and other contextual factors:

> For me in the work that I do there's two extremes … . One is, I'm doing a job, part of that job is around my personal sexual identity and personal commitment to a community, but none the less it is a job. The other extreme is I'm doing something for my community and around my identity and I happen to get paid for it, which is nice. (Nick, London)

As their sexuality was often seen to be key to their professional role, outreach workers had more than one way in which to relate to others. This could create profound conflicts with service users, colleagues and other professionals. For example, an emphasis on sexuality could lead to sexual harassment from managers, accusations of being 'over involved' in the work by colleagues and over-identification with service users. This kind of tension is something that has also been highlighted in HIV-related care. For example:

> there are significant numbers of people who fall into this broad category of 'professionals' and who are also people living with HIV or AIDS. Inevitably, they sometimes feel caught in the middle when the interests of these two groups fail to coincide … there are many who clearly identify more closely with people living with the virus than with the policy and procedural imperatives of the organizations by whom they are employed.
>
> (MacLachlan 1992:443)

Too strong an emphasis on shared identifications can lead to workers being seen as over-involved, and therefore unprofessional (Purtilo 1993). For example, Hanmer and Statham (1993) in an article on the relationship between women social workers and their female clients, describe how although they often experience links with them, they are not encouraged to recognise these for fear of over-identification or over-involvement. Professionalism has traditionally been seen to be about creating distance from others:

> An important element of the professional–client relationship, it is proposed, is that of 'mystification': professionals promote their services as esoteric. They create dependence on their skills and reduce the areas of knowledge and

experience they have in common with their clients. In this way they increase the 'social distance' between themselves and their clients, and so gain increasing autonomy.

(Williams, J. 1993:8–9)

This situation has been compounded by expectations of 'objectivity' as an element of professional practice. This causes problems for the caring professions in particular because their work involves a degree of involvement which others would see as undermining their professionalism. Whatever the professional doctrine, accounts of everyday practice show that many professionals do use personal experience when working (Deverell and Sharma 2000; Wakeling 1993). As ideas about professionalism change, in some cases it is becoming more acceptable to introduce more personal and passionate elements into professional roles (Whyte 1996). For those involved in community based work, an understanding of professionalism which embraces such things as the importance of knowledge gained through personal experience, workers' political commitment, and community involvement (see also Ussher 1993), may make the adoption of a professional identity sit more comfortably for many. However, it still raises issues about how much the personal experiences, values and feelings of an individual worker should influence what is done.

Emotion work

As outlined in Chapter 1, there is growing recognition of the ways in which emotions are used as an institutional resource. For example, O'Brien (1994) argues that in order to control encounters, and promote health messages and behaviours, nurses use various forms of emotional labour. These include establishing trust and confidence, comforting patients and providing support. Bolton suggests that the use sociologically of the term 'emotion labour' undermines the complexity of different forms of emotion management that may be used in a single occupation. She highlights four different types of emotion management:

> presentational (emotion management according to general social 'rules'), philanthropic (emotion management given as a 'gift'), prescriptive (emotion management according to organisational/professional rules of conduct) and pecuniary (emotion management for commercial gain). The categorisation of various forms of emotion management ... help to display its multi-faceted nature.

(O'Brien 2000:214)

In this study outreach workers used different kinds of emotion management with clients, colleagues and managers. Emotional resources were used to make contact, establish empathy, encourage trust, carry out counselling, manage encounters and effect change within organisational environments. Workers also placed great emphasis on managing their own emotions in terms of self-presentation, detachment and self-disclosure. This included managing both their own and others' anger and sexual feelings in order to maintain appropriate boundaries.

One of the issues created by the use of personal creativity and emotional resources in service jobs is the personal cost to workers themselves. Several writers have reported that where workers carry out a considerable amount of emotion management, they may experience burnout or problems in switching off from their work role. As Hochschild notes:

> Trainers take it as their job to attach to the trainee's smile an attitude, a viewpoint, a rhythm of feeling that is, as they often say, 'professional!' This deeper extension of the professional smile is not always easy to retract as the end of the workday, as one worker in her first year at World Airways noted: 'Sometimes I come off a long trip in a state of utter exhaustion, but I find I can't relax. I giggle a lot, I chatter, I call friends. It's as if I can't release myself from an artificially created elation that kept me "up" on the trip.'
>
> (Hochschild 1983:4)

In this study too, workers talked about finding it difficult to switch off from work and discussed the impact this had on their own social and sexual lives. Interestingly, many workers reported positive emotional effects on themselves and their personal lives through the skills they had learned in work. For example, some reported being more confident and self-assertive. However, this was tempered with stories about becoming emotionally detached or exhausted. Many interviewees spoke of the need for emotional support themselves to enable them to continually support others. It was emotional needs such as these that could put workers in a vulnerable position:

> If you're feeling great and you're feeling OK, and you're out working, you feel: 'right we don't have any problem with boundaries.' It's when you're not feeling so great, you've had a hard time, you're looking for a bit of soft and fluffy you know you want somebody to just take you home and give you a big cuddle. You need that sort of intimacy with somebody, anybody sometimes.
> (Edward, Midlands)

Where a job demands high emotional input, support and supervision become vital. This is particularly the case for lone community based workers who at times can feel a responsibility to solve everyone's problems.

Sexual skills

As outlined in Chapter 1, some writers have started to write more specifically about the use of sexual skills in certain occupations. Adkins (1992), who has carried out work on women in the tourist industry, suggests that men rarely have to engage in sexual work, and uses this as an argument to support her view that gender needs to be placed more centrally within the analysis of sexuality in organisations. However, a focus on gender, although helpful in addressing the sexual labour women undertake, neglects important issues relating to sexuality. This study showed that some men do use sexual skills in work. In the case of outreach work this was done to make contact, build trust, challenge organisational homophobia and to develop more effective campaigns. More specifically, workers used their appearance and body to make contact with service users:

> If you walk around as an outreach worker and adopt quite a professional manner then people will tend to blend back into the trees ... (*laughs*). And you don't make any contact. But if you walk along as if you're cruising ... that's what attracts them. (Derek, London)

Although men's use of sexual or flirtation strategies to encourage the use of a service may not yet be common, it seems likely that as more men become involved in service occupations their use of such techniques may become more frequent.

The effective use of sexual skills involves deploying them in a way that avoids unwanted harassment or sexual advances. Interpersonal interaction is often sexualised when the product or subject of work is of a sexual nature. This means interactions have to be carefully managed to ensure that sex does not actually take place. Abraham's (1994) study of lingerie selling in a department store showed that in order to ensure that the sexual fantasies used to sell women's underwear were not acted upon, the interactions between male customers and assistants, and female customers and fitters or sellers, had to be kept asexual. The methods of interaction used to draw boundaries here involved not being naked, avoiding close contact with flesh and using medical language (1994:11). In nursing too, the potentially sexual character of some nurse–patient interactions has to be managed. Rhodes (1994b), for example, mentions that because nurses have intimate contact with strangers, this may make them seem available and willing sexual partners. For this reason, Lawler (1993) writes that to spare the embarrassment of patients, and prevent unwanted sexual advances, nurses may try to 'professionalise the encounter' when bathing patients or carrying out other intimate procedures.

As outlined in Chapters 5 and 6, because the place and nature of outreach work did not immediately communicate their professional role, interviewees' relationship with clients often involved a process of negotiation whereby they established the limits of the relationship. This was felt to be less of an issue in more structured interactions in offices where the boundaries of the relationship with workers were likely to be more clearly understood by service users. However, in PSEs workers had to use various strategies to manage potentially sexual interactions. The fact that they were undertaking innovative work was important in this respect. For example, one man described how he had worked in social spaces before, as a barman. However, here he had not found difficulties in maintaining sexual boundaries as his recognised and accepted position as a barman provided clear expectations both to himself and customers about the extent of his role.

The limits of shared identity

> The way we work and the way [other projects] are working has proved that
> you know as out gay men you can do a lot ... . But what does happen is that
> means you do choose your target groups ... . Approaching men who may be
> married, have no contact with the gay world at all ... how comfortable do they
> feel to be approached by a very out gay men who wants to talk? ... The whole
> point of going cottaging half the time is that people aren't going to talk to you,
> they don't want to know about your life, or what you do ... I'm not completely
> sure about the appropriateness of us, as very out gay men, working in that
> field. I think maybe there's room for other people to do that work, um more, you
> know, straight looking straight-acting or whatever ... . So that's my quandary
> about it. As far as the skills as gay men [go], I think they're vital in clubwork
> and scene work, without them you wouldn't last a minute. (Andrew, North)

Studies of outreach work have shown that there are limits to whom gay men can
contact through their displays of sexuality (Daly and Horton 1993; Davis *et al.*
1991; Prout and Deverell 1995; Van Reyk 1990). It is for reasons such as this that
Broadhead *et al.* (1995) suggest that outreach workers are best working with those
most like themselves. This is supported by the recent work of Flowers and Hart
(1999) who, in a study of gay clubs in Glasgow, found that because the gay scene
is so divided in terms of cliques, effective peer education outreach should involve
'social network-specific, indigenous outreach workers' (1999:94) (though interestingly not necessarily men).

In the present study, having a similar sexuality to service users was felt by many
of the male interviewees to engender trust, understanding and empathy which was
crucial to the success of outreach. However, workers identified one of the problems with the emphasis on sexuality was that they did not necessarily have similar
experiences to the men they worked with, even though they may have the same
sexual identity. Indeed, several workers discussed how emphasising their sexual
identity could cause difficulties because it rendered invisible the other skills they
had, created assumptions about their knowledge and experience, and minimised
differences between gay men.

Advocates of the view that gay men are the best candidates to undertake work
with other gay men often downplay the differences between gay men. Gatter
(1999) argues that this is a result of pursuing political goals. It is important to
recognise that having a shared sexuality does not necessarily mean that outreach
workers have a thorough understanding of the diversity of all gay men's needs. It is
also true that successful HIV prevention with gay men can be achieved by those
with a different sexuality. Certainly all four women interviewed as part of this
study had been actively involved in outreach work with gay and bisexual men. As
one of them described her experiences:

> I asked a few of the men just to gauge what they thought about a woman being
> there, and they all had no issue about it. They said it was normal sort of thing

.... Nobody made any sort of negative comments ... I mean one in particular said: 'Well I have no issue about you being here as long as you don't sit on my face!' *(laughs)* ... . But that was it really that was all I had. And I think perhaps they assumed that there are a lot of women that work within, I don't know gay sexual health, doctors' surgeries, any sort of actual services really, so there was no issue around that at all. (Sarah, London)

Some of the strongest criticism about professional HIV prevention workers and boundaries has come from people who have not undertaken full time outreach work (e.g. King 1993b). Their emphasis on the importance of peer education amongst gay men and the need for a shared sexuality successfully to carry out work seems at odds with the experiences of those directly involved in HIV prevention. In recent years there has been a growing recognition amongst those undertaking HIV work with gay men that identity alone is not a sufficient qualification for quality HIV prevention and can downplay the other skills needed. Even within organisations such as GMFA, there has been a growing recognition that gay volunteers require interpersonal skills and training to carry out successful motivational interviewing in outreach. As Harris notes:

This training will require volunteers to master a defined body of knowledge, skills and attitudes.

(Harris 1999:4)

Peer educators require excellent social skills and a range of health promotion competencies in addition to being able to flirt or empathise with gay men. Shepherd *et al.* (1999) argue that because peer educators are often more comfortable as information providers rather than agents of attitude and behaviour change, there is a need to identify the full range of skills needed to undertake HIV prevention work. This may mean different roles for paid HIV workers:

The increasing complexity of gay and bisexual men's responses to the epidemic requires equally sophisticated health promotion interventions, and it is clear that we are now asking far more from peer educators than ever before. What is not clear is whether it is realistic to recruit and train peer educators to fully address the agenda for HIV prevention with gay and bisexual men.

(Shepherd *et al.* 1999:168)

Those interviewed for this study stressed that outreach work is not something that all gay men can do but requires training, support and interpersonal skills. This emphasis partly related to their need to gain credibility and respect for their role; however, it also recognised the realities of the skills needed for this type of HIV prevention work.

A further issue relating to the emphasis on using shared experience is that employing gay male workers can be seen as a way of community based working in itself, regardless of the actual methods used. As Brager and Specht (1973) note, the use of methods to encourage community participation can vary greatly from consultation to direction and ownership. So while some see community based working as trying to empower and enable people to develop their own health promotion initiatives (Miller 1994; Prout and Deverell 1995), others feel that as part of a community they have the knowledge to define the needs of service users themselves. These distinctions are extremely important as they have a great impact on the way in which work is carried out. An over-reliance on personal experience can be potentially very damaging as workers' own experiences and needs are often different from those of other gay and bisexual men, many of whom do not prioritise HIV prevention (see also Kotarba and Lang 1986). Indeed, as outreach workers become professionalised they may lose touch with the very social group they are employed to work with (Broadhead *et al.* 1995).

As highlighted in Chapter 2, the experiences of both researchers and outreach workers suggest that shared identities do not necessarily lead to automatic alliances and can hide power relationships. Although the emphasis on shared characteristics may enrich relationships, it is naive to focus purely on their utility as this neglects issues of power and difference which occur within communities. It is important to address the limits of shared experience as well as the benefits.

Home and Work

Bailey (2000) has argued that the private sphere is taking on increased cultural importance. Interestingly, this comes at a time when it could be argued that less and less of people's experience is truly private. However, the desire to maintain some separation between different parts of their life was clearly expressed by the outreach workers in this study. Despite the integrated nature of their work and personal lives, many of those interviewed still hankered after a backstage where they could relax and be their private self. This meant putting effort into constructing and maintaining areas of their lives separate from work. Their experiences highlighted the fact that although the public–private construct is too simplistic, it still provides a powerful organising frame.

One of the reasons why workers in this study found difficulties in keeping personal and work life separate, was because of the small and networked nature of the gay and bisexual communities in which they worked (see also Ryan 1995). It was the close integration of their social and work networks which led them to feel that the ideal of separating home and work was impossible:

> You're a gay man in your social life, you're also a gay man professionally ... and there never seems to be this let off of something completely different from what you do ... you never really leave your job at work in some respects. You know, you feel as if your life is being paid for by the health authority.
> (Richard, Midlands)

Those living and working in the same community often find this leads to a blurring of boundaries between work and personal life. Interestingly, the experience of living and working closely with the same group of people is seen to be a growing phenomenon in the UK, in part related to the increase in working hours for those in full employment:

> Britain is a nation in love with its colleagues. We don't just work with them, we eat with them, drink with them, play sport with them and have sex with them ... . The reasons for this have much to do with modern living. According to national statistics, at least 75 per cent of the population is working 30 hours or more a week, which doesn't leave a lot of time for anything after work.
>
> (Tucker 2000:294–5)

This experience of integration underlines the impact of work on different aspects of people's lives, particularly where occupational and social networks overlap. In her study of clergy wives Finch (1983a:44) describes three main ways that work can spill over into non-work life: being mentally at work most of the time; via the replication of patterns of working relationships; and by escaping from work and the need to counter its effects. She argues that these responses vary with particular occupations and the spatial relationship between home and work. The outreach workers in this study mentioned all of the effects described by Finch. However, they also talked more specifically about the impact of work on their friendship networks and personal sex lives.

The influence of work on sexual activity has rarely been referred to in any detail in the literature. Occasionally there are references to the impact of work on home and family life, or a sentence or two addressing an issue such as the effect of work-related stress on sex. However, in this study where individuals were working in sexualised environments in a sexually defined community there was a lot of discussion about the impact of work on their sex lives. Interviewees talked in detail about experiences such as being restricted in their choice of sexual partners, or feeling responsible for safer sex because their professional identity continued into their personal relationships. In this way their experiences directly questioned the writing of sociologists who have seen sex as separate to, or as an escape from, work. Despite the complaints of some outreach workers in the study, it is clear that it is not only gay men whose sexual behaviour and relationships are subject to work-related restrictions and organisational ideals about public and private boundaries. There appears to be increasing regulation and questioning of sexual boundaries in many occupations:

> It is as traditional a part of office life as the broken photocopier and that rough bit under a desk that ladders your tights. Now, however, some companies have banned the quick fumble behind the filing cabinet. Marks and Spencer, Royal Bank of Scotland, HSBC, Nat West and some Civil Service departments have made romance in the office a sackable offence ... other firms have gone further, deciding that any relationship between colleagues, even one conducted out of hours is a breach of contract ... the British work the longest hours in Europe. If we don't meet our partner at work, we'll all be sat in on a Friday

night weeping into our take-away pizzas … . Employers reap the benefits of the long-hours culture … . For them now to ban the one way most of us find love is ludicrous and cruel.

(Turner 2000:30)

Luxton has argued that having sex is acquiring increased significance for people as it becomes more identified with: 'leisure activities, popularity and personal expression' (1980:60). If this is the case, then there may be increasing resistance from workers to such regulation as we saw from some individuals in this study. Certainly some of the dilemmas concerning sexual relationships and work which interviewees described are now being discussed more openly in other occupations.

The ways in which people manage their personal and work lives is an issue little explored in the literature. Outreach workers clearly felt an expectation that they should have a separate personal life, and manage it in a way that would not undermine their professional reputation (Horobin 1983, Paterson 1983). However, having a job that explicitly used their personal experiences, and working and living in the same community, many found this ideal unrealistic. The exploration of their struggles shows the effort required to create different public and private spheres through boundary making and highlights the fact that the ideal of separate spheres is not so easily achieved in practice.

Sexual identity, community and boundaries

It's about trying to make your own sexuality and your sex life separate from work really which is the difficulty. (George, North)

Participation in the gay community is for many gay men a central way of expressing sexual identity. A focus on the importance of shared social spaces is not to deny other links gay men may have, for example through politics, friendship or work or to suggest that all gay men's social lives are the same. That said, the importance of the commercial gay scene both as a place of community and identity and as a space for exploring sexuality should not be underestimated. As Adam has observed:

central to the emergence of the post-war gay and lesbian worlds have been the commercial venues which created public spaces for homosexually interested people. These commercial settings have not only facilitated the development of the modern gay world, but have influenced its content.

(Adam 1992:175)

Eisenstadt and Gatter's (1999) more recent research on social and sexual networks in London has shown that bars are a central institution in gay life, and that bars and clubs are by far the most frequent sites for gay men to meet sexual partners. The significance of such venues for many gay men helps to explain the reactions of some workers in this study to adopting boundaries that prevented them from using gay bars or clubs in their own time if they also worked in them. Many of the outreach workers in small towns, where there may only be one gay venue, felt that there were no other places in which they could pursue their own sex and leisure interests. As described in Chapters 5 and 6, the centrality of sexual participation for some men meant that guidelines which restricted where they could have sex were experienced as repressing their own sexuality. It is important to understand that for these men not having sex was not just experienced as limiting opportunities for sexual gratification, but was about giving up ties to community and friendship.

The study showed a range of feelings amongst those interviewed, with those gay men who were younger or who socialised most on the gay scene experiencing more conflicts between their work and personal lives. For those workers who saw having sex with other men as central to their own sexual identity, keeping boundaries was often much harder. This was clearly contrasted in the interviews with women; the fact that they did not participate sexually in the community in which they worked was often explicitly identified as a factor that helped in boundary maintenance. In fact, issues around boundaries seemed most troublesome for single gay men who wanted to use the places they worked in to meet partners themselves. This necessitated developing clear ideas about who was 'out of bounds':

> I think everybody has a right to have sex ... and that's why it's quite good to have clear guidelines about who is and who isn't a client. (Sean, North)

> we see things we fancy we want them, just like every other gay man on the scene. It's a matter of just being able to compartmentalise when you have them, if you can have them, and so on ... there are right places and right times, and I think that's fair enough. (Edward, Midlands)

Workers' understanding of their relationship with service users played a key role in their definition of appropriate professional conduct and its translation into the process of boundary making. For some the regulation of sexual activity through boundary making was seen as a necessary part of the job, whereas for others it represented repression and homophobia. Different understandings about the purpose of HIV prevention work, and the best form of relationship to have with service users, sometimes led to profound disagreements over the need for boundaries. For example, those who saw their primary role as providing life-saving information to their peers had very different ideas about having sex with service users to those who saw their role as being paid to provide health promotion and counselling. For some men, it was the focus on relating to other men as peers ('we're all gay'), which led them to question traditional ideas about the power relationships between professionals and clients to their activities. Furthermore, some interviewees argued that being in a gay culture, which emphasised the positive nature of sex, meant that if you did not express anger at, or problems with, maintaining sexual boundaries, other workers did not see you as 'a proper gay man'. It was this emphasis on the positive right to have sex that was seen by some workers

as having led to a denial amongst some gay men's workers that sex could be difficult or abusive:

> There's something very gendered about the way, about the kind of very secure
> way that gay men would argue on it somehow. There's very little sense of an
> experience of sex ever being negative which I think is very male. I mean it
> isn't true about men, but it's very socially masculine isn't it? Really. You
> rarely get any sense that, that sex is bad really, other than well you might get
> this disease from it. But there's very little sense of sex being about power over
> other people even in subtle or blatantly crude and abusive ways really. (Tim,
> London)

Overall, outreach workers' experiences highlight the need for a more sophisticated approach to understanding sexual boundaries. There is clearly a need to distinguish between the different kinds of relationship workers have with service
users. Certainly, it seems extreme to view a worker having sex with someone as a
form of abuse when they have only given them a condom. However, in more
involved counselling-type encounters the situation is obviously quite different.
This study demonstrated that making sexual boundaries is a far broader issue than
just preventing abuse by workers and that discussions in this area need to include a
range of situations and experiences. A better appreciation of the nuances involved
in HIV prevention work of this kind would also help those having to make and
keep these different sexual boundaries.

The new professionalism and work–life balance

> If the physics of our universe is revealing the primacy of relationships, is it
> any wonder that we are beginning to reconfigure our ideas about management
> in relational terms? ... We are refocusing on the deep longings we have for
> community, meaning, dignity, and love in our organizational lives. We are
> beginning to look at the strong emotions that are part of being human, rather
> than segmenting ourselves (love is for home, discipline is for work) or believ-
> ing that we can confine workers into narrow roles, as though they were cogs in
> the machinery of production. As we let go of the machine models of work, we
> begin to step back and see ourselves in new ways, to appreciate our whole-
> ness, and to design organizations that honor and make use of the totality of
> who we are.
>
> (Wheatley 1994:12)

Ideas about sex, work and professionalism change over time. Influences as
diverse as quantum physics (relationships and self-organising systems), neurosci-
ence (emotional intelligence), feminism (personal experience and relationships)
and poetry (bringing emotion and spirituality into work) are just some of the current sources shaping ideas about management and professionalism. These ideas

both form, and are formed by, the experiences of individual workers. In the West the growth of long working hours, competitive pressure and job insecurity is leading to a questioning of the privileging of work over other areas of life. Furthermore, increasing openness and media interest in the private lives of public figures is questioning the relationship between private lives and work or professional roles. This climate means that issues of professionalism and boundary making are becoming more relevant to a wider range of occupations than HIV prevention outreach.

The interconnections between different aspects of people's lives is clearly demonstrated in outreach workers' experiences. Many of the links between work and personal lives they described can be seen to apply to occupations more generally. For example, taking work home, using personal experience, or dealing with crises which affect the amount of time available for leisure. As Lyon argues, for most employees the influence of work continues outside of it:

> For some people, occupation and the work role that goes with it may be simply a way of earning a living, and of little intrinsic importance. For many, however, the work role is crucial and can give meaning to life outside work. Our occupation can determine our standard of living, our sense of self-esteem, the degree to which we can exercise power and autonomy in our life and our physical and mental health. Even if we thoroughly dislike our work it can have far-reaching effects on our life.
>
> (Lyon 1993:234)

The growing recognition of the links between work and other parts of life has led to a new emphasis on what is being called work–life balance:

> The key stress that is most difficult to monitor is the balancing act between work and life, between the demands of a hyper competitive work environment and domesticity … . A number of studies have shown that people work better when they are happy at home. In addition, they tend to stay in their jobs … . As a result initiatives have been devised to teach people how to manage work and life.
>
> (Appleyard 2000)

In the UK, a new independent body 'Employers for Worklife balance' comprising twenty-two companies (including Lloyds, TSB, BT, Asda, Unilever, and Littlewoods) has begun a dialogue with the government to tackle what they see as the urgent need for more flexible working practices and 'family friendly' policies (*Diversity Challenge* 2000:5). This interest in work–life balance is not simply altruistic; companies believe they will be better able to recruit and keep the best workers by making these changes. Furthermore, they aim to reduce the amount of absenteeism and sick leave caused by stress and to improve morale. There is also a recognition that work itself is changing. For example, as more employees begin to work from home new types of worker–manager relationships and boundaries are needed:

> Anyone who exchanges the daily commute for a more flexible way of working will find this leads to big changes in all areas of their lives. The balance between work and personal life, especially if they opt to work from home, will never be the same again … . One of the main issues is ensuring strict boundaries between work and family time.
>
> (Cooper 2000)

Although these kinds of job are quite different to outreach, it is interesting that similar issues relating to the management of boundaries between different parts of life occur. It could be argued that those working from home are also having to learn how to live and work in the same spaces. Tips on how to develop personal and work boundaries are already starting to appear in the popular press and in company magazines. Although various practical suggestions are made, for example having a separate office space, a separate telephone line, getting dressed and setting fixed working hours (Cooper 2000; Dawson 2000) individuals' management of time, friends, family relationships and feelings of guilt or isolation are seen to be key:

> Autonomy can work only if it goes hand in hand with self-control, trustworthiness, and conscientiousness. And as people work less 'for the company' and more for themselves, emotional intelligence will be required to maintain the relationships vital for workers' survival.
>
> (Goleman 1999:314)

Emotional intelligence refers to the ability to manage emotions, recognise feelings and motivate the self. It is the combination of these skills with technical expertise and ability that Goleman (1999) argues is crucial to the success of both individuals and organisations:

> The rules for work are changing. We're being judged by a new yardstick: not just by how smart we are, or by our training and expertise, but by how well we handle ourselves and each other … . These rules have little to do with what we were told was important in school; academic abilities are largely irrelevant to this standard. The new measure takes for granted having enough intellectual ability and technical know-how to do our jobs; it focuses instead on personal qualities, such as initiative and empathy, adaptability and persuasiveness … . In a time with no guarantees of job security, when the very concept of a 'job' is rapidly being replaced by 'portable skills', these are prime qualities that make and keep us employable. Talked about loosely for decades under a variety of names, from 'character' and 'personality' to 'soft skills' and 'competence', there is at last a more precise understanding of these human talents, and a new name for them: emotional intelligence.
>
> (Goleman 1999:3–4)

While this may seem far away from the world of outreach, we can see many of the dilemmas outreach workers faced reflected in such organisational developments. For example, relying on their intuition and judgement, working in less managed work spaces, managing their own and others' feelings and expectations and keeping time for a private life. Furthermore, the growing emphasis in many organisations on the importance of managing relationships and the desire for increased personal passion at work means that employers are beginning to demand new skills and qualities from their employees, those that in the past may have been seen to be of a more personal nature. This stress on personal skills and experiences rather than expert knowledge has close parallels with the qualities outreach workers felt had led to their employment. It seems likely that new understandings about being professional will emerge with these changes in workers' roles and qualifications. Indeed, learning from the outreach workers interviewed also suggests that this increasing emphasis on personal qualities and emotion work will require new measures to reduce workers' emotional stress and the incidence of burnout.

The relevance of outreach workers' experiences to new debates about the nature and organisation of work is also apparent in the move in many occupations towards less hierarchical organisations, a greater emphasis on casual dress and more flexible working practices. These changes mean that more workers are having to learn to operate in environments where there are fewer visible signs that communicate their professional role. As in outreach, this will mean individual workers having both to take more responsibility for managing boundaries and to find ways of behaving appropriately and accountably without formal organisational structures and close supervision. This emphasis on self-management will require new kinds of skills and support.

This study emerged from a recognition of the tensions those in HIV prevention outreach work were having to manage between the realities of their working lives and more traditional ideas about the nature of work and professionalism. This community based and sex-related occupation was seen to be unusual, challenging both organisations and social theorists in their thinking about the nature and management of work. It is hoped that the detailed exploration of outreach workers' experiences has provided greater insight into the realities of this type of HIV prevention, enabling both workers and managers better to appreciate the dilemmas and difficulties involved in such frontline work. Many of the questions raised in this book about the meaning of professionalism, the pain and pleasure in emotion work and the management of boundaries between home, sex and work are being asked more generally by workers in a range of organisations. Therefore, whilst the experiences of outreach workers remain specific, elements of their struggles, desires and beliefs about work have clear applicability to thinking and practice in a much wider range of occupations.

Notes

1 Sex, work and professionalism: theoretical issues

1 Interestingly, in the 1990s the rise of women working full time in the UK, coupled with the longest working hours in Europe, can be seen as a spur to the increasing availability and use of domestic services (*The Trend Letter* 1997). With no one at home to be doing the laundry, cooking, cleaning and repairs, new services are emerging to cater for these increasingly visible needs.

2 Halford *et al.* (1997) report that in the banks they studied it was openly acknowledged that men's home lives were central to their career prospects. Although it is less likely these days that men will have to be married with children before they are made managers there still seems to be a preference for men to fit this mould.

3 When talking informally to people about this study, I found that they would often relate tales about boundary issues they had experienced. For example, colleagues in their first lecturing jobs would discuss having to make decisions about whether or not to socialise with students. They often found it hard, having recently graduated and still very much identifying with the student community, to develop a distanced role as a lecturer. Deciding whether to socialise in the Students Union, dealing with sexualised comments on their appearance, or issues related to fancying students were often raised at dinner parties or in the pub. Like those I interviewed, many complained that they received little managerial or organisational guidance on how to deal with such situations.

3 HIV prevention, gay communities and outreach work

1 As Hart notes, some of the techniques and behaviours used in safer sex had been practised long before, notably by female sex workers (1993). Depending on the definition used, much contraceptive practice could also be seen as a form of safer sex. Indeed, many of the issues of trust, negotiation and long term motivation seem similar.

2 Useful, though at times partial, summaries of the development of HIV prevention for gay men in Britain can be found in Davies *et al.* 1993 and King 1993a.

3 It is not strictly correct to polarise the voluntary and statutory sector responses, as those from voluntary organisations began to move into newly created HIV prevention posts, and those in the statutory sector often sat on the boards of voluntary organisations or provided support and advice (Bennett and Ferlie 1994).

4 The government cancelled a national sex survey, which it had commissioned, and which was considered vital to help plan appropriate HIV prevention (Whitehead 1989). It is reported that it was the then prime minister's own distaste that was a major factor in this decision (Garfield 1994). The research was eventually successfully completed through funding from the Wellcome Foundation.

5 A further point to note is that because of the lack of other health and social services designed for gay men, HIV services often take on more than their remit because they have identifiable expertise and contacts with gay men. This puts a large burden on these projects to address more than HIV.

4   Sex, sexuality and work

1   The display of sexual material can be seen as an attempt to 'homosexualise' the workplace in a similar manner to that described by Westwood (1984), whereby women sought to 'feminise' the factory.

2   Rules related to not having sex with colleagues were rarely codified in organisational guidelines; however, three interviewees discussed guidelines about not having sexual relationships with staff or colleagues. These were mainly related to those they had a managerial relationship with. A few other interviewees refused to have sex with colleagues as a personal boundary.

3   At least three of the men interviewed were not out about their sexuality to their families, and as such could not tell them their job titles. This did not seem to be uncommon, as other interviewees talked about workers they knew who were only 'out' at work. This is the reverse of many gay men's experiences who may be out to families and friends but not at work (Burke 1994).

5   The impact of work on personal life

1   Of course, the portrayal of sex in these terms is also what makes realistic safer sex strategies difficult to design for sex educators (Holland *et al.* 1989; 1990).

6   Boundary work

1   Curtis and Hodge suggest one ethical guideline for judging whether a behaviour is going beyond boundaries is to judge: 'How comfortable would the provider be if this action was reported in the paper?' (1995:6)

2   This is a phenomenon that has also been noted by Cruikshank (1989) who found that single women community development workers experienced the most severe burnout. They tended to pour all their energies into work, and did not have the emotional support and escape mechanisms of their married colleagues. Importantly, they were also expected to take on more weekend work because they were single.

3   Something of the variety in service users reactions to workers can be seen in the following quote: 'On a professional level you get "I don't need one because I've got my partner", or "You're too late"; I mean that's always a bit of a deadener, a bit of a conversation stopper. Or "I don't need one of those", or "Do you fancy showing me how to use one of those?", "Does this pack come with a man?", "What are you doing at eleven o'clock?", "Never mind the condom, what are you doing at eleven o'clock?", "Let me know when you've got a night off", "When are you going to show me how to use it?" (*laughs*) .... You name it. "Why isn't there more lubricant in these packs?" .... "This condom's not big enough for me" .... There's all sorts of things. Or "Ger her over there she needs ten." That's another one (*laughs*). In the end a lot of it's meant in good humour.' (Edward, Midlands)

7   Professionalism and sexual identity

1   Although outreach workers borrowed ideas about professionalism derived from therapeutic helping relationships, in reality their experiences were often quite different. For example, they go out providing services, their places of work are public settings, the length of client contact is usually shorter and the nature of some service user relationships is quite ambiguous.

2   While knowledge through contact, participation and observation was also brought to the work by women, for example by being part of the lesbian and gay community, by having gay friends, or through direct learning from gay men, women rarely emphasised their experience in the same way.

3   Specifically, the desires of a mainly young, white, middle class, fashionable and out group of gay men, whose social lives revolve around the many gay bars, restaurants and shops in Soho, London (see Mort 1996).

4   This interviewee spoke a lot about not feeling valued in the work and being an easy target for criticism for being a woman in a 'gay men's business'. She felt that it was very rare that gay men

would stand up for her even though she felt she spent a lot of time supporting them and challenging homophobia (see also Gorna 1996).

5   It is an interesting twist that in gay men's work the characteristics associated with 'professionals' are those more usually seen as the antonyms of professional: amateurish, incapable, incompetent, inefficient, inept, inexperienced, unpolished, unqualified, unskilled, untrained (*Collins English Dictionary* 1990:559). Such criticisms have been levelled particularly at middle aged, heterosexual women who are felt not to understand gay culture and are seen to have no knowledge about working appropriately with gay men.

6   In an interview in the gay press the general manager of GMFA when asked 'Do you ever pick up volunteers?' answered (presumably half-jokingly) 'Yes, it's GMFA policy and part of my job description.' (*Boyz* 1995b).

7   A good exploration of many of the concerns that workers have expressed about this model of working can be found in Miller 1993 (see also McPherson 1993).

8   Interestingly, at times HIV workers have been seen as a clique of their own, being labelled the AIDS Mafia or AIDS Clergy, by other gay men (Simpson 1995:90).

Bibliography

Abraham, H.E. (1994) 'The social construction of women's sexuality in a department store', paper presented to the British Sociological Association Conference 1994, College of St Mark and St John (mimeo).

Abramson, A. (1992) 'Between autobiography and method. Being male, seeing myth and the analysis of structures of gender and sexuality in the Eastern interior of Fiji', in D. Bell, P. Caplan and W.J. Karim (eds) *Gendered Fields, Women, Men and Ethnography*, London: Routledge.

Adam, B.D. (1992) 'Sex and caring among men: impacts of AIDS on gay people', in K. Plummer (ed.) *Modern Homosexualities: Fragments of Lesbian and Gay Experience*, London: Routledge.

Adkins, L. (1992) 'Sexual work and the employment of women in the service industries', in M. Savage and A. Witz (eds) *Gender and Bureaucracy*, Oxford: Blackwell.

Adkins, L. and Lury, C. (1994) 'The cultural and the sexual and the gendering of the labour market', paper presented to the British Sociological Association Conference 1994, University of Lancaster (mimeo).

Agar, M.H. (1980) *The Professional Stranger: An Informal Introduction to Ethnography*, London: Academic Press.

Aggleton, P., Jordan, S., Stoakes, P. and Wilton, T. (eds) (1990) *Outreach Work With Men Who Have Sex With Men*, Bristol: Southmead Health Authority/The Health Education Authority.

Aggleton, P., Weeks, J. and Taylor-Laybourn, A. (1993) 'Voluntary sector responses to HIV and AIDS: A framework for analysis', in P. Aggleton, P. Davies and G. Hart (eds) *AIDS: Facing The Second Decade*, London: Falmer Press.

Allgeier, E. (1984) 'The personal perils of sex researchers: Vern Bullough and William Masters', *SIECUS Report* 12(4): 16–19.

Altman, D. (1986) *AIDS and the New Puritanism*, London: Pluto Press.

—— (1988) 'Legitimation through disaster: AIDS and the gay movement', in E. Fee and D. Fox (eds) *AIDS The Burdens of History*, London: University of California Press.

—— (1989) 'AIDS and the reconceptualization of homosexuality', in D. Altman, H. Van den Boogaard, L. Borghi, I. Foeken, M.E. Hunt, A. Van Kooten Niekerk, M. Van Lieshout, T. Van der Meer, G. Menard, J. Schippers, R. Trumbach, M. Vicinus, C.S. Vance, J. Weeks, S. Wieringa and M. Wittig (eds) *Homosexuality, which Homosexuality?* London: Gay Men's Press.

—— (1993) 'Expertise, legitimacy and the centrality of community', in P. Aggleton, P. Davies and G. Hart (eds) *AIDS: Facing The Second Decade*, London: Falmer Press.

—— (1994) *Power and Community. Organizational and Cultural Responses to AIDS*, London: Taylor & Francis.

Anderson, W., Hickson, F. and Stevens, C. (1994) *Health Purchasing, HIV Prevention and Gay Men*, London: Health Education Authority.

Andrews, M. (1991) *Lifetimes of Commitment: Aging, Politics, Psychology*, Cambridge: Cambridge University Press.

Annetts, J. and Thompson, B. (1992) 'Dangerous activism?', in K. Plummer (ed.) *Modern Homosexualities: Fragments of Lesbian and Gay Experience*, London: Routledge.

Appleyard, B. (2000) 'Work', *The Sunday Times Magazine*, 25 June: 41–7.

Arning, B. (1996) 'Introduction', in *Brenda and Other Stories, Art and HIV and You*, Walsall Museum and Art Gallery, Walsall.

Ashton, J. and Seymour, H. (1988) *The New Public Health*, Milton Keynes: Open University Press.

Bailey, J. (2000) 'Some meanings of "the private" in sociological thought', *Sociology*, 34(3): 381–401.

Bailey, W. (1995) 'The importance of HIV prevention programming to the lesbian and gay community', in G.M. Herek and B. Greene (eds) *AIDS, Identity and Community, the HIV Epidemic and Lesbians and Gay Men*, London: Sage.

Baker, J. and Craig, M. (1990) 'Management committees as one model of local accountability: the lessons we can learn from our experience', paper given to Roots and Branches: a Winter School on Community Development and Health, March 1990 (mimeo), Milton Keynes: Open University.

Barrett, M. and McIntosh, M. (1982) *The Anti-social Family*, London: Verso.

Bartos, M., McLeod, J. and Nott, P. (1993) 'Meanings of sex between men', study conducted by the Australian Federation of AIDS Organisations for the Commonwealth Department of Health, Housing, Local Government and Community Services.

Baum, F. (1988) 'Community-based research for promoting the new public health', *Health Promotion* 3(3): 259–68.

Baxter, J. and Western, M. (1998) 'Satisfaction with housework: examining the paradox', *Sociology* 32(1): 101–21.

Beattie, A. (1991) 'Knowledge and control in health promotion: a test case for social policy and social theory', in J. Gabe, M. Calnan and M. Bury (eds) *The Sociology of the Health Service*, London: Routledge.

BBC (1996) 'Eternal Light', Soho Stories, 4 November, BBC2.

Bedell, G. (1991) 'The Westminster boss as sex object: extremely unlikely', *Independent*, 20 October: 2.

Bennett, C. and Ferlie, E. (1994) *Managing Crisis and Change in Health Care*, Buckingham: Open University Press.

Berridge, V. (1992) 'AIDS, the media and health policy', in P. Aggleton, P.M. Davies and G. Hart (eds) *AIDS: Rights, Risk and Reason*, London: Falmer Press.

BOSS (Birmingham Outreach Safe Squad) (1994) 'Birmingham Outreach Safe Squad, first report' (mimeo), Birmingham: South Birmingham Community NHS Trust.

Bloor, M. (1995) *The Sociology of HIV Transmission*, London: Sage.

Blundy, A. and Katz, I. (1994) 'Who's a pretty boy then?', *Guardian*, 21 January: 2–3.

Bolton, R., Vincke, J. and Mak, R. (1994) 'Gay baths revisited', *GLQ: A Journal Of Lesbian & Gay Studies* 1(3): 255–73.

Bolton, S.C (2000) 'Mixed feelings: emotion management in a caring profession', in N. Malin (ed.) *Professionalism, Boundaries and the Workplace*, London: Routledge.

Bonell, C. (1996) *Outcomes in HIV Prevention, Report of a Research Project*, London: The HIV Project.

Boy George with Bright, S. (1995) *Take it Like a Man: The Autobiography of Boy George*, London: Sidgwick and Jackson.

Boyz (1995a) 'The art of cruising men', *Boyz*, 18 November: 79.

—— (1995b) 'Probe with Martin', *Boyz*, 20 May.

Brah, A. (1992) 'Difference, diversity and differentiation', in J. Donald and A. Rattansi (eds) *'Race', Culture and Difference*, London: Sage.

Brager, G. and Specht, H. (1973) *Community Organising*, Columbia: Columbia University Press.

Brewis, J. and Kerfoot, D. (1994) 'Selling our 'selves'? Sexual harassment and the intimate violations of the workplace', paper presented to British Sociological Association Conference 1994 (mimeo).

Broadhead, R., Heckathorn, D., Grund, J.C., Stern, L.S. and Anthony, D.L (1995) 'Drug users versus outreach workers in combatting AIDS', *International Journal of Drug Policy* 6(4): 274–88.

Brodsky, A. (1989) 'Sex between patient and therapist: Psychology's data and response', in G. O'Gabbard (ed.) *Sexual Exploitation in Professional Relationships*, Washington DC: American Psychiatric Press.

Brookman, J. (1993) 'Conduct code for campus love affairs', *Times Higher Educational Supplement*, 15 January, 1054: 2.

Bryant, C.D. (ed.) (1974) *Deviant Behaviour: Occupational and Organisational Bases*, Chicago: Rand McNally.

Bryson, I. (1994) personal communication.

Burke, M. (1994) 'Dissident identities: The case of the gay police officer', paper given to BSA Conference 1994, Psychology Department, Brunel University (mimeo).

Burrell, G. (1984) 'Sex and organisational analysis', *Organisation Studies* 5(2): 97–118.

Burton, S. (1989) 'Safer sex ads: are they too little too late?', *Pink Paper*, 11 February, 59: 2.

Cain, R. (1994) 'Managing impressions of an AIDS service organization: into the mainstream or out of the closet?', *Qualitative Sociology* 17(1): 43–61.

Campbell, D. (1988) 'AIDS: patient power puts research on trial', *New Scientist*, 12 November: 26–7.

—— (1989) 'Well done, Capital AIDS!', Body Matters Special Report, *Pink Paper* 20 January, 376: 4.

Capital Gay (1988a) 'Better six years late than never', *Capital Gay*, 2 December, 371: 9.

—— (1988b) 'Angry storm over "dangerous" ads', *Capital Gay*, 9 December, 372: 9.

—— (1988c) 'The HEA must think again!', Body Matters, *Capital Gay*, 9 December, 372: 4.

—— (1989) 'Government promotes safer gay sex', *Capital Gay*, 10 February, 379: 11.

Carter, S. (1995) 'The "gay handshake" no longer exists', *Pink Paper*, 23 June.

Cavendish, R. (1982) *Women on the Line*, London: Routledge.

CDC (1981) *Morbidity and Mortality Weekly Reports*, 5 June.

Chadwick, H. (1994) *Effluvia Catalogue*, London: Serpentine Gallery.

Clayton, R. (1993) 'A practical role for health service health promotion agencies?', *Health Education Journal* 52(2): 96–8.

Clifford, J. and Marcus, G.E. (eds) (1986) *Writing Culture: The Poetics and Politics of Ethnography*, London: University of California Press.

Cockburn, C. (1983) *Brothers: Male Dominance and Technological Change*, London: Pluto Press.

Cohen, N. (1992) 'Out in the undergrowth', *Independent on Sunday*, 15 March: 3.

Collins English Dictionary (1990) London: Collins.

Collinson, D. L. and Collinson, M. (1993) 'Sexuality in the workplace: the domination of men's sexuality', in J. Hearn, D.L. Sheppard, P. Tancred-Sheriff and G. Burrell (eds) *The Sexuality of Organization*, London: Sage.

Comer, L. (1974) *Wedlocked Women*, Leeds: Feminist Books.

Cooper, C.L. (2000) 'Make time to work and relax', *The Sunday Times, The New Work How the Information Revolution Can Change Your Life Supplement*, 7 May 7: 2

Cotterill, P. (1992) 'Interviewing women, issues of friendship, vulnerability and power', *Womens' Studies International Forum* 15(5–6): 593–606.

Coward, R. (1994) 'And then she kissed me ...', *Observer People*, 23 January: 21.

Coxon, T. (1988) 'Review essay: Social science and AIDS', *Sociology of Health and Illness* 10(4): 609–13.

Craib, I. (1995) 'Some comments on the sociology of the emotions', *Sociology*, February, 29(1): 151–9.

Crompton, R. and Sanderson, K. (1990) *Gendered Jobs and Social Change*, London: Unwin Hyman.

Cruikshank, J. (1989) 'Burnout: an issue among Canadian community development workers', *Community Development Journal* 24(1): 40–54.

Curtis, L. and Hodge, M. (1995) 'Boundaries and HIV-related care management', *Focus: A Guide to AIDS Research and Counselling* 10(2): 5–6.

Daily Telegraph (1996) 'Pandering to gay lust', Editorial comment, *Daily Telegraph*: 17.

Daly, J. and Horton M. (1993) 'Take prevention to the people', *AIDS Action* June–August, 21: 2–3.

Davidoff, L. and Westover, B. (eds) (1986) *Our Work, Our Lives, Our Words*, Basingstoke: Macmillan Education.

Davies, C. (1996) 'The sociology of professions and the profession of gender', *Sociology* 30(4): 661–79.

Davies, P.M., Hickson, F.C.I., Weatherburn, P. and Hunt, A.J. (1993) *Sex, Gay Men and AIDS*, London: Falmer Press.

Davis, M.D., Klemmer, U. and Dowsett, G.W. (1991) *Bisexually Active Men and Beats: Theoretical and Educational Implications*, Sydney: AIDS Council for New South Wales and Macquarie University AIDS Research Unit.

Dawson, C. (2000) 'First, take your pyjamas off', *Sunday Times, The New Work How the Information Revolution Can Change Your Life Supplement*, 7 May: 4–5.

Day, N.E. *et al.* (1996) *Incidence and Prevalence of Other Severe HIV Disease in England and Wales for 1995–9: Projections Using Data to end of 1994*, Communicable Diseases Report 6, London: Public Health Laboratory Service.

de Croy, D. (1990) 'Workshop on working in the public environment', in P. Aggleton, S. Jordan, P. Stoakes and T. Wilton (eds) *Outreach Work With Men Who Have Sex With Men*, Bristol: Southmead Health Authority/The Health Education Authority.

Devaney, K. (1991) 'Mining a world apart', in V.J. Siedler (ed.) *The Achilles Heel Reader, Men, Sexual Politics and Socialism*, London: Routledge.

Deverell, K. (1993) 'Using participant observation in sauna outreach', *Practicing Anthropology* Fall 15(4): 44–8.

Deverell, K. and Bell, J. (1993) 'Some thoughts on being straight women in a men who have sex with men project', Keele University: Department of Sociology and Social Anthropology (mimeo).

Deverell, K. and Prout, A. (1995) 'Sexuality, identity and community: reflections on the MESMAC project', in P. Aggleton, P. Davies and G. Hart (eds) *AIDS: Safety, Sexuality and Risk*, London: Taylor and Francis.

Deverell, K. and Rooney, M. (1995) *Using Sexually Explicit Materials for Safer Sex Work with Gay Men*, London: The HIV Project.

Deverell, K. and Sharma, U. (2000) 'Professionalism in everyday practice: issues of trust, experience and boundaries', in N. Malin (ed.) *Professionalism, Boundaries and the Workplace*, London: Routledge.

DHSS/Welsh Office (1987) *AIDS: Monitoring Response to the Public Education Campaign*, London: Department of Health and Social Security.

Dillner, D. (1996) 'Sheets of shame', *Guardian*, 30 April: 10.

Dingwall, R. (1979) *The Social Organization of Health Visiting*, Beckenham: Croom Helm.

Diversity Challenge (2000) *Unilever Employee Magazine*, Issue 9, July, Dorset: Broglia Press.

Dockrell, M. (1993) 'Cum with rubbers!', *F***Sheet*: November, 2: 1.

—— (1994) 'More fucking boyfriends', *F***Sheet*: March, 5: 5–7.

—— (1995) 'A tramp on the Heath', *F***Sheet*: 5–6.

—— (1996) 'The morning after the night before', *F***Sheet*, May, 24: 1–2.

DoH (1992) *The Health of the Nation: A Strategy for Health in England*, London: Department of Health.

—— (1993) *The Health of the Nation: Key Area Handbook: HIV/AIDS and Sexual Health*, London: Department of Health.

Duck, S. (1986) *Human Relationships: An Introduction to Social Psychology*, London: Sage.

Duncombe, J. and Marsden, D. (1995) '"Workaholics" and "whingeing women": theorising intimacy and emotion work: the last frontier of gender inequality?', *Sociological Review* 43(1): 150–70.

Eden, J. (1996) 'Gays' loos get a safe sex squad', *Daily Star*, 3 August.

Edwards, N. (1995) 'Police and gay group tackle condom tree', *Pink Paper*, 1 September: 6

Edwards, T. (1994) *Erotics and Politics: Gay Male Sexuality, Masculinity and Feminism*, London: Routledge.

Eisenstadt, K. and Gatter, P. (1999) 'Coming together: social networks of gay men and HIV prevention', in P. Aggleton, G. Hart and P.M. Davies (eds) *Families and Communities Responding to AIDS*, London: UCL Press.

Elshtain, J.B. (1981) *Public Man, Private Woman*, Oxford: Martin Robertson.

Engels, F. (1972) *The Origin of the Family, Private Property and the State*, New York: Pathfinder Press.

Evans, B.A., McLean, K.A., Dawson, S.G., Teece, S.A., Bond, R.A., MacRae, K.D. and Thorp, R.W. (1989) 'Trends in sexual behaviour and risk factors for HIV infection among homosexual men, 1984–7', *British Medical Journal* 6668(298): 215–8.

Fahey, T. (1995) 'Privacy and the family: conceptual and empirical reflections', *Sociology* November, 29(4): 687–703.

Fetterman, D. (1991) 'A walk through the wilderness. Learning to find your way', in W.B. Shaffir and R.A. Stebbins (eds) *Experiencing Fieldwork, An Inside View of Qualitative Research*, London: Sage.

Field, N. (1992) 'Take-over bids and monopolies: HIV and the gay community', *Mainliners Newsletter*, August–September, 25/26: 1–3.

Finch, J. (1983) *Married to the Job, Wives' Incorporation in Men's Work*, London: Allen and Unwin.

—— (1993) ' "It's great to have someone to talk to": Ethics and politics of interviewing women', in M. Hammersley (ed.) *Social Research, Philosophy, Politics and Practice*, London: Sage.

Fineman, S. (1991) 'Organising and emotion', paper given at Towards A New Theory of Organisations Conference, University of Keele, April 1991, School of Management, University of Bath: Bath (mimeo).

Fisher, J. (1996) *1995 Hampstead Heath Report*, London: Gay Men Fighting AIDS.

Fisher, T.D. (1989) 'Confessions of a closet sex researcher', *Journal of Sex Research* 26(1): 144–7.

Fitzpatrick, R., Boulton, M. and Hart, G. (1989) 'Gay men's sexual behaviour in response to AIDS', in P. Aggleton, P. Davies and G. Hart (eds) *Social Representations, Social Practices*, London: Falmer Press.

Fitzpatrick, R., Dawson, J., Boulton, M., McLean, J. and Hart, G. (1991) 'Social psychological factors that may predict high risk sexual behaviour in gay men', *Health Education Journal* 50(2): 63–6.

Fitzpatrick, R., McLean, J., Boulton, M., Hart, G. and Dawson, J. (1990) 'Variation in sexual behaviour in gay men', in P. Aggleton, P. Davies and G. Hart (eds) *AIDS: Individual, Cultural and Policy Dimensions*, London: Falmer.

Flowers, P. and Hart, G. (1999) 'Everyone on the scene is so cliquey', in P. Aggleton, G. Hart and P.M. Davies (eds) *Families and Communities Responding to AIDS*, London: UCL Press.

Forbes, S. (2000) 'Should "baregobbling" still be called safer sex?', *F***Sheet* April, 55: 2.

Forgacs, (ed.) (1988) *A Gramsci Reader: Selected Writings 1916–1935*, London: Lawrence and Wishart.

Foster, J. (1988) 'Impact of the AIDS epidemic on the gay political agenda', in I.B. Corless and M. Pittman-Lindeman (eds) *AIDS: Principles, Practices and Politics*, London: Hemisphere.

Foucault, M. (1979) *Discipline and Punish*, Harmondsworth: Penguin.

—— (1981) *The History of Sexuality, Volume 1, An Introduction*, trans. Robert Huxley, London: Lane.

Fowler, D. and Hardesty, D. (1994) *Others Knowing Others. Perspectives on Ethnographic Careers*, London: Smithsonian Institution.

Francoeur, R. (1996) '*Sex, Priests and Power: Anatomy of a Crisis* by A.W. Richard Snipe', book review *Journal of Sex Research* 33(1): 77–8.

Freidson, E. (1983) 'The theory of professions: state of the art', in R. Dingwall and P. Lewis (eds) *The Sociology of the Professions*, London: Macmillan.

—— (1984) 'The changing nature of professional control', *Annual Review of Sociology* 10: 1–20.

Friedman, J. and Mobilia Boumil, M. (1995) *Betrayal of Trust: Sex and Power in Professional Relationships*, Westport: Praeger.

*F***Sheet* (1999) 'Drugs, saunas and SM: Microcommunities take off', *F***sheet* 47: 1–3.

Gans, H.J. (1968) 'The participant-observer as human being: observations on the personal aspects of fieldwork', in H.S. Becker, B. Geer, D. Reisman and R.S.Weiss (eds) *Institutions and The Person: Papers Presented to Everett C. Hughes*, Chicago: Aldine Publishing Company.

Garfield, S. (1994) *The End of Innocence: Britain in the Time of AIDS*, London: Faber and Faber.

Gatter, P. (1993) 'Anthropology and the culture of HIV/AIDS voluntary organisations', in P. Aggleton, P. Davies and G. Hart (eds) *AIDS: Facing the Second Decade*, London: Falmer Press.

—— (1999) *Identity and Sexuality, AIDS in Britain in the 1990s*, London: Cassell.

Gechtman, L. (1989) 'Sexual contact between social workers and their clients', in G. O'Gabbard, (ed.) *Sexual Exploitation in Professional Relationships*, Washington DC: American Psychiatric Press.

Glazer, N. (1990) 'The home as workshop: women as amateur nurses and medical care providers', *Gender and Society* 4(4): 479–99.

Gledhill, R. (1996) 'Runaway RC bishop has son aged 15', *The Times* 20 September: 1.

Goleman, D. (1999) *Working with Emotional Intelligence*, London: Bloomsbury.

Gonsiorek, J.C. (1995) *Breach of Trust: Sexual Exploitation by Health Care Professionals and Clergy*, Thousand Oaks: Sage.

Goode, W.J. (1957) 'Community within a community: the professions', *American Sociological Review* 22: 194–200.

Gorna, R. (1996) *Vamps, Virgins and Victims. How can women fight AIDS?*, London: Cassell.

Gorna R. and Harris, R. (1996) 'The end of innocence: THT re-buffs attack', *The Trust* Newsletter: 12.

Goss, D. and Adam-Smith, D. (1994) 'Framing difference: sexuality, AIDS and organization', paper presented to British Sociological Association Conference 1994, University of Central Lancashire, Portsmouth: Portsmouth Business School (mimeo).

Gowler, D. and Legge, K. (1978) 'Hidden and open contracts in marriage', in R. Rapoport and R.N. Rapoport (eds) *Working Couples*, London: Routledge and Kegan Paul.

Grant, L. (1992) 'The lid on the id', *Independent on Sunday*, 10 May: 26.

Greenwood, E. (1957) 'Attributes of a profession', *Social Work*, July, 2: 45–55.

Grey, A. (1993) *Speaking of Sex*, London: Cassell.

Griffin, C. (1991) 'The researcher talks back. Dealing with power relations in studies of young people's entry into the job market', in W.B. Shaffir and R.A. Stebbins (eds) *Experiencing Fieldwork, An Inside View of Qualitative Research*, London: Sage.

Griffiths, A. (1995) 'Services for gay men', *Agenda*, June–August: 6–7.

Gutek, B. (1989) 'Sexuality in the workplace: key issues in social research and organizational practice', in J. Hearn, D.L. Sheppard, P. Tancred-Sheriff and G. Burrell (eds) *The Sexuality of Organization*, London: Sage.

Halford, S., Savage, M. and Witz, A. (1997) *Gender, Careers and Organisations, Current Developments in Banking, Nursing and Local Government*, London: Macmillan.

Hall, M. (1989) 'Private experiences in the public domain: lesbians in organizations', in J. Hearn, D.L. Sheppard, P. Tancred-Sheriff and G. Burrell (eds) *The Sexuality of Organization*, London: Sage.

Hall, S. (1990) 'Cultural identity and diaspora', in J. Rutherford (ed.) *Identity, Community, Culture, Difference*, London: Lawrence and Wishart.

Hammersley, M. (1992) 'On feminist methodology', *Sociology* 26(2): 187–206.

Hammersley, M. and Atkinson, P. (1993) *Ethnography Principles in Practice*, London: Routledge.

Hanmer, J. and Statham, D. (1993) 'Commonalities and diversities between women clients and women social workers', in J. Walmsley, J. Reynolds, P. Shakespeare and R. Woolfe (eds) *Health Welfare and Practice: Reflecting on Roles and Relationships*, London: Open University Press/Sage.

Haraway, D. (1990) 'A manifesto for cyborgs: science, technology, and socialist feminism in the 1980s', in L.J. Nicholson (ed.) *Feminism/Postmodernism*, London: Routledge.

Harries, S. (1989) 'No sex research please, we're British', *Pink Paper*, 91: 8.

Harris, O. (1981) 'Households as natural units', in K. Young, C. Walkowitz and R. McCullagh (eds) *Of Marriage and the Market. Women's Subordination Internationally and its Lessons*, London: Routledge and Kegan Paul.

Harris, Q. (1999) 'Tools for talking heads', *F***Sheet*, December, 53: 1–4.

Harrison, T. (1994) 'Gay men and sexual health', *Agenda*, March–May: 5.

Harrison, T. (ed.) (1943) *Mass Observation War Factory: A Report*, London: Victor Gollancz.

Hart, A. (1992) *Purchasing Power? An Ethnographic Study of Men Who Buy Sex in Alicante, Spain*, DPhil, Trinity, Oxford.

—— (1993) 'Participation, observation and sex research', paper presented to ASA Decennial Conference 1993, University of Keele: Department of Sociology and Social Anthropology (mimeo).

Hart, G. (1993) 'Safer sex: a paradigm revisited', in P. Aggleton, P. Davies and G. Hart (eds) *AIDS: Facing The Second Decade*, London: Falmer Press.

—— (1995) 'The evaluation of behavioural interventions in gay men: will evidence based on prevention become the norm?', paper given to HIV Behavioural Interventions Conference, Royal Society of Medicine, June, Glasgow: MRC Medical Sociology Unit.

Hearn, J. and Parkin, W. (1987) *Sex At Work: The Power and Paradox of Organisation Sexuality*, Brighton: Wheatsheaf Books.

Hearn, J., Sheppard, D.L., Tancred-Sheriff, P. and Burrell, G. (eds) (1989) *The Sexuality of Organization*, London: Sage.

Henriksson, B. and Mansson, S. (1992) 'Sexual negotiations, an ethnographical study of men who have sex with men', paper presented to AIDS and Anthropology Group, Culture, Sex Behaviour and AIDS, Amsterdam, Department of Social Work, University of Gothenburg (mimeo).

Hickson, F. (1995) 'Unsafe sex goes on', *Pink Paper*, 20 October.

Hickson, F., Davies, P., Wych, G. and Project SIGMA (1993) 'Brief encounters: characteristics and sources of casual sexual partners among gay and bisexual men', in P. Aggleton, P. Davies and G. Hart (eds) *AIDS: Facing The Second Decade*, London: Falmer Press.

Hickson, F. and Keogh, P. (1995) 'The reality of sex is not a PR exercise', *Pink Paper*, 17 November 1995: 7.

Hickson, F. and Maguire, M. (1996) 'Thinking it through: a booklet for gay men, an example of collaborative working bridging research and HIV prevention targeting gay men', paper presented to Building Bridges Conference, The Institute of Education, London.

Hochschild, A. (1983) *The Managed Heart: The Commercialisation of Human Feeling*, Berkeley: University of California Press.

Holland, J., Ramazanoglu, C. and Scott, S. (1990) 'AIDS: from panic stations to power relations: sociological perspectives and problems', *Sociology* 25(3): 499–518.

—— (1989) 'Managing risk and experiencing danger. Tensions between government AIDS education policy and young women's sexuality', paper presented to the British Sociological Association Conference, Plymouth Polytechnic, 21–23 March (mimeo).

Homans, H. and Aggleton, P. (1988) 'Health education, HIV infection and AIDS', in P. Aggleton and H. Homans (eds) *Social Aspects of AIDS*, London: Falmer Press.

Horobin, G. (1983) 'Professional mystery: the maintenance of charisma in general medical practice', in R. Dingwall and P. Lewis (eds) *The Sociology of the Professions*, London: Macmillan.

Howard, J. (1995) 'You don't have to be mad to work here ...', *Boyz*, 22 July: 18.

Hunt, A.J., Davies, P.M., Weatherburn, P., Coxon, A.P.M. and McManus, T.J. (1991) 'Changes in sexual behaviour in a large cohort of homosexual men in England and Wales 1988–9', *British Medical Journal* 2 March, 302: 505–6.

Hunt, A.J., Weatherburn, P., Hickson, F.C.I., Davies, P.M., McManus, T.J. and Coxon, P.M. (1993) 'Changes in condom use in gay men', *AIDS Care* 5(4): 439–49.

Independent (1992a) 'Office sex pests "get off lightly"', *Independent*, 11 January.

—— (1992b) 'Companies "are failing to tackle sexual harassment"', *Independent*, 7 March.

Ishiguro, K. (1990) *The Remains of the Day*, London: Faber and Faber.

Jeffreys (1996) 'Women who use sex to sell', *Marie Claire*.

Jenkins, J. (1990) 'Privates on parade', *New Statesman and Society*: 10–11.

Johnson, M. (1983) 'Professional careers and biographies', in R. Dingwall and P. Lewis (eds) *The Sociology of the Professions*, London: Macmillan.

Johnson, T. (1981) *Professions and Power*, London: Macmillan.

Jones, B. (1972) 'Sex in the office', *National Times*, 12 June.

Jones, C. and Causer, G. (1994) 'Learning the rules of the game: sexuality, equality and power in the technical workplace', paper presented to the British Sociological Association Conference (mimeo).

Kanter, R.M. (1977) *Men and Women of the Corporation*, New York: Basic Books.

Kellner, P. (1991) 'One in six women sexually harassed', *Independent*, 20 October, 91: 1.

Kennett, S. (1995) 'Negative closets', *Capital Gay*, 3 March.

Keogh, P. and Holland, P. (1999) 'Observing the rules: an ethnographic study of London's cottages and cruising areas', in P. Aggleton, G. Hart and P.M. Davies (eds) *Families and Communities Responding to AIDS*, London: UCL Press.

King, E. (1991) 'Safer sex revolutionaries', *Pink Paper*, 14 December, 205: 9.

—— (1993a) *Safety in Numbers*, London: Cassell.

—— (1993b) 'Beating boundaries', *Pink Paper*, 17 September, 295: 14.

—— (1995) 'Stab in the dark', *Pink Paper*, 1 September: 8.

—— (2000) 'Revenge of the poison penis', *F***Sheet*, April, 55: 1–3.

King, E., Rooney, M. and Scott, P. (1992) *HIV Prevention for Gay Men: A Survey of Initiatives in the UK*, London: North West Thames Regional Health Authority.

Kingman, S. (1994) 'Quality control for medicine', *New Scientist*, 17 September: 22–6.

Kinsman, G. (1997) 'Managing AIDS organizing: 'consultation', 'partnership', and the national AIDS strategy', in W.K. Carroll (ed.) *Organizing Dissent: Contemporary Social Movements in Theory and Practice*, 2nd edition, Aurora, Ontario: Garamond Press.

Kleinman, S. (1991) 'Field-worker's feelings. What we feel, who we are, how we analyse', in W.B. Shaffir and R.A. Stebbins (eds) *Experiencing Fieldwork, An Inside View of Qualitative Research*, London: Sage.

Knights, D. and Morgan, G. (1991) 'Organisation theory consumption and the service sector', paper presented to Towards a New Theory of Organizations Conference, University of Keele, 3–5 April 1991, Manchester: Manchester School of Management (mimeo).

Kotarba, J. and Lang, N. (1986) 'Gay lifestyle change and AIDS: preventive health care', in D. Feldman and T. Johnson (eds) *The Social Dimensions of AIDS, Method and Theory*, London: Praeger.

Kowalewski, M.R. (1988) 'Double stigma and boundary maintenance: how gay men deal with AIDS', *Journal of Contemporary Ethnography*, 17(2): 211–28.

Kramer, L. (1983) 'I,112 and counting', *The New York Native*: 1.

—— (1990) *Reports From the Holocaust, the Making of an AIDS Activist*, London: Penguin.

Kulick, D. and Wilson, M. (1995) *Taboo: Sex, Identity and Erotic Subjectivity in Anthropological Fieldwork*, London: Routledge.

Larson, M.S. (1977) *The Rise of Professionalism: A Sociological Analysis*, London: University of California Press.

—— (1990) 'In the matter of experts and professionals, or how impossible it is to leave nothing unsaid', in R. Torstendahl and M. Burrage (eds) *The Formation of Professions, Knowledge, State and Society*, London: Sage.

Lasch, C. (1995) *Haven in a Heartless World: The Family Besieged*, New York: WW Norton and Co.

Latour, B. (1990) 'Drawing things together', in M. Lynch and S. Woolgar (eds) *Representation in Scientific Practice*, Cambridge, Mass: MIT Press.

Lawler, J. (1993) *Behind the Screens. Nursing, Somology and the Problem of the Body*, London: Churchill Livingstone.

Laws, S. (1990) *Issues of Blood: The Politics of Menstruation,* Hampshire: Macmillan Press.

Leslie, T. (1993) 'Safer sex drive sparks death threat', *Pink Paper*, 30 July, 288: 1.

Lindenbaum, S. (1991) 'Anthropology rediscovers sex', *Social Science Medicine* 33(8): 865–6.

Lippert. J. (1977) 'Sexuality as consumption', in J. Snodgrass (ed.) *For Men Against Sexism: A Book of Readings*, Albion, CA: Times Change Press.

Littlejohn, R. (1996) 'Even I couldn't make this up', *Daily Mail*, 2 August.

Lyon, K. (1993) 'Why study roles and relationships?', in J. Walmsley, J. Reynolds, P. Shakespeare and R. Woolfe (eds) *Health Welfare and Practice: Reflecting on Roles and Relationships*, London: Open University Press/Sage.

Luxton, M. (1980) *More Than a Labour of Love: Three Generations of Women's Work in the Home*, Toronto: Womens Press.

MacDonald, K. (1992) *Professional Project and Cultural Context*, Occasional Papers in Sociology and Social Research, Department of Sociology, University of Surrey.

—— (1995) *The Sociology of the Professions*, London: Sage.

MacLachlan, J. (1992) 'Managing AIDS: a phenomenology of experiment, empowerment and expediency', *Critique of Anthropology* 12(4): 433–56.

MacLeod, D. (1993) 'Code demands dons declare affairs with students', *Independent*, 16 January.

Maslanka, H. (1993) 'Women volunteers at GMHC', in C. Squire (ed.) *Women and AIDS*, London: Sage

Maslen, G. (1995) 'Sex codes for safe conduct', *Times Higher Educational Supplement* 29 December: 5.

Maupin, A. (1990) *Babycakes*, London: Black Swan.

May, C. (1992) 'Individual care? Power and subjectivity in therapeutic relationships', *Sociology* 26(4): 589–602.

May, C., Dowrick, C. and Richardson, M. (1996) 'The confidential patient: the social construction of therapeutic relationships in general medical practice', *Sociological Review* 44(2): 187–204.

McElhinny, B. (1994) 'An economy of affect objectivity, masculinity and the gendering of police work', in A. Cornwall and N. Lindisfarne (eds) *Dislocating Masculinity*, London: Routledge.

McNestry, M. and Hartley, M. (1995) *Developing a Local Response: Gay and Bisexual Men's Needs in Relation to HIV and AIDS*, Bexley: Bexley and Greenwich Health.

McPherson, M. (1993) 'Tearing down boundaries', *Pink Paper*, 1 October: 297.

Meikle, J. (1992) 'No sex please, we're lecturers', *Guardian* 15 May.

Meldrum, J. (1993) 'Squaring up to an epidemic', *Pink Paper* 20 June: 12.

Mezzone, J. (1996) 'Linking research and practice: a provider's perspective', in K. Deverell (ed.) *Building Bridges, Linking Research and Primary HIV Prevention*, Conference Report, London: NAM Publications.

Miller, D. (1993) 'Peer education: the answer to our prayers, or an overrated fad?', paper given to HIV Prevention With Gay and Bisexual Men Conference, Durham 25 July, MESMAC Tyneside, Newcastle-upon-Tyne (mimeo).

—— (1994) letter in *Gay Times*, December.

Mort, F. (1996) *Cultures of Consumption: Masculinities and Social Space in Late Twentieth Century Britain*, London: Routledge.

Murray, S. (1992) 'Components of gay community in San Francisco', in G. Herdt (ed.) *Gay Culture in America: Essays from the Field*, Boston: Beacon Press.

Narayan, K. (1993) 'How native is a "native" anthropologist?', *American Anthropologist* 95: 671–86.

Needham, A. (2000) 'Whatever happened to AIDS?', *The Face* 3(39): 164–8.

Nickolay, C. (1991) 'Computer games', in V.J. Seidler (ed.) *The Achilles Heel Reader. Men, Sexual Politics and Socialism*, London: Routledge.

O'Brien, M. (1994) 'The managed heart revisited: health and social control', *Sociological Review* 42(3): 393–413.

O'Gabbard, G. (ed.) (1989) *Sexual Exploitation in Professional Relationships*, Washington DC: American Psychiatric Press.

Oakley, A. (1974) *The Sociology of Housework*, London: Martin Robertson.

—— (1981) 'Interviewing women. A contradiction in terms?', in H. Roberts (ed.) *Doing Feminist Research*, London: Routledge and Kegan Paul.

Ottawa Charter for Health Promotion (1986) *Ottawa Charter for Health Promotion*, Health & Welfare Canada, Canadian Public Health Association.

Padgug, R.A. and Oppenheimer, G.M. (1992) 'Riding the tiger: AIDS and the gay community', in E. Fee and D.M. Fox (eds) *AIDS the Making of a Chronic Disease*, Oxford: University of California Press.

Parkin, W. and Green, L. (1994) 'Sexuality and residential care research in progress', paper presented at the British Sociological Association Conference 1994 (mimeo).

Parsons, quoted in Edgell, S. (1980) *Middle Class Couples: A Study of Segregation, Domination and Inequality in Marriage*, London: Allen and Unwin.

Paterson, A. (1983) 'Becoming a judge', in R. Dingwall and P. Lewis (eds) *The Sociology of the Professions*, London: Macmillan.

Patton, C. (1985) *Sex and Germs: The Politics of AIDS*, Boston: South End Press.

—— (1990) *Inventing AIDS*, London: Routledge.

—— (1990) 'What science knows: formations of AIDS knowledges', in P. Aggleton, P. Davies and G. Hart (eds) *AIDS: Individual, Cultural and Policy Dimensions*, London: Falmer.

Patton, D. (1995) 'Can sex spell success?', *Girl About Town*, 6 November: 1170.

Phoenix, V. (1995) 'Dressing down', *Pink Paper*, 9 June.

Pink Paper (1988) 'Beeb news blunder', *Pink Paper* 8 December, 52: 1.

—— (1991) '26 blunders', *Pink Paper*, 2 November, 199: 1.

—— (1994a) 'HEA reviews safer sex campaigns', *Pink Paper*, 22 April: 2.

—— (1994b) 'Government vetoes AIDS ads', *Pink Paper*, 4 February, 313: 3.

—— (1994c) 'Sex on tap', *Pink Paper* 11 November.

—— (1994d) 'AIDS worker attacked', *Pink Paper* 29 July, 338: 3.

—— (1995a) 'Fair weather friends', *Pink Paper*, 1 December: 17.

—— (1995b) 'Gay safer-sex worker forced out of home', *Pink Paper*, 21 July.

Plummer, K. (1988) 'Organizing AIDS', in P. Aggleton and H. Homans (eds) *Social Aspects of AIDS*, London: Falmer Press.

—— (1995) *Telling Sexual Stories: Power, Change and Social Worlds*, London: Routledge.

Pollert, A. (1981) *Girls, Wives and Factory Lives*, London: Macmillan.

Pope, (1989) 'Teacher–student sexual intimacy', in G. O'Gabbard (ed.) *Sexual Exploitation in Professional Relationships*, Washington DC: American Psychiatric Press.

Positive Nation (1995) 'Positive men deserve more from GMFA', *Positive Nation*, November, 2: 28.

Powell, A. and Elkins, T. (1993) *Cambridge MESMAC Project 1989–1993, Evaluation Report*, Cambridge: Cambridge Health Promotion and AIDS Services.

Power, L. (1993) 'Diary', *Pink Paper* 21 March: 269.

Prentice, A. (1994) *Cottaging and Cruising Project in South West London*, London: Wandsworth, Merton and Sutton and Croydon Health Authorities and South West Thames Regional Health Authority.

Pringle, R. (1988) *Secretaries Talk: Sexuality, Power and Work*, London: Verso.

—— (1989) 'Bureaucracy, rationality and sexuality: the case of secretaries', in J. Hearn, D.L. Sheppard, P. Tancred-Sheriff and G. Burrell (eds) *The Sexuality of Organization*, London: Sage.

Prout, A. and Deverell, K. (1995) *Working with Diversity – Building Communities: Evaluating the MESMAC Project*, London: Health Education Authority.

Purtilo, R. (1993) 'Meaningful distances', in J. Walmsley, J. Reynolds, P. Shakespeare and R. Woolfe (eds) *Health, Welfare and Practice: Reflecting on Roles and Relationships*, London: Open University Press/Sage.

Rechy, J. (1978) *The Sexual Outlaw*, London: WH Allen.

Rhodes, P. (1994a) 'Race of interviewer effects in qualitative research', *Sociology* 28(2): 547–59.

—— (1994b) '"Nice girls don't do that". Gender, pollution and professional boundaries in the performance of intimate procedures for patients with continence problems', paper presented to British Sociological Association Conference, University of Central Lancashire, York: Social Policy Research Unit (mimeo).

Rhodes, T., Holland, J. and Hartnoll, R. (1991) *Hard to Reach or Out of Reach? An Evaluation of an Innovative Model of HIV Outreach Health Education*, London: Tuffnell Press.

Robinson, D. (1973) *Patients, Practitioners and Medical Care: Aspects of Medical Sociology*, London: William Heinemann.

Rooney, M. and Scott, P. (1992) 'Working where the risks are: health promotion interventions for gay men and other men who have sex with men in the second decade of the HIV epidemic', London: Health Education Authority (mimeo).

Rosica, T.C. (1995) 'AIDS and boundaries: instinct versus empathy', *Focus: A Guide to AIDS Research and Counseling* 10(2): 1–4.

Roy, D. (1974) 'Sex in the factory: informal heterosexual relations between superiors and work groups', in C.D. Bryant (ed.) *Deviant Behaviour: Occupational and Organisational Bases*, Chicago: Rand McNally.

Rubin, G. (1992) 'Thinking sex: notes for a radical theory of the politics of sexuality', in C.S. Vance (ed.) *Pleasure and Danger, Exploring Female Sexuality*, London: Pandora Press.

Rueschmeyer, D. (1983) 'Professional autonomy and the social control of expertise', in R. Dingwall and P. Lewis (eds) *The Sociology of the Professions*, London: Macmillan.

Rust, P.C. (1993) ' "Coming out" in the age of social constructionism: sexual identity formation among lesbian and bisexual women', *Gender and Society* 7(1): 50–77.

Rutter, P. (1991) *Sex in the Forbidden Zone. When Men In Power – Therapists, Doctors, Clergy, Teachers and Others – Betray Women's Trust*, London: Mandala Press.

Ryan, L. (1990) 'Reflections on the AIDS panic', *Living Marxism* January: 15–19.

—— (1995) ' "Going public" and "watching sick people": The clinic setting as a factor in the experiences of gay men participating in AIDS clinical trials', *AIDS Care* 7(2): 147–58.

Sandfort, T. (1995) 'HIV/AIDS prevention and the impact of attitudes towards homosexuality and bisexuality', in G.M. Herek and B. Greene (eds) *AIDS, Identity and Community, the HIV Epidemic and Lesbians and Gay Men*, London: Sage.

Saunders, P. (1990) *A Nation of Homeowners*, London: Unwin Hyman.

Schneider, B.E. (1986) 'Coming out at work: Bridging the private–public gap', *Work and Occupations* 13(4): 463–87.

Schover, L. (1989) 'Sexual exploitation by sex therapists', in G. O'Gabbard (ed.) *Sexual Exploitation in Professional Relationships*, Washington DC: American Psychiatric Press.

Schramm-Evans, Z. (1990) 'Responses to AIDS, 1986–1987', in P. Aggleton, P. Davies and G. Hart (eds) *AIDS: Individual, Cultural and Policy Dimensions*, London: Falmer.

Scott, P. (1993) 'Beginning HIV prevention work with gay and bisexual men', in B. Evans, S. Sandberg and S. Watson (eds) *Healthy Alliances in HIV Prevention*, London: Health Education Authority.

—— (1995a) 'Question and answer', Raccoon's Column *F***Sheet* June, 16: 6–8.

—— (1995b) *Pink Paper*, 15 September.

Secrett, D. (1991) 'Homogenised', in V.J. Seidler (ed.) *The Achilles Heel Reader. Men, Sexual Politics and Socialism*, London: Routledge.

Seidler, V.J. (1991) 'Recreating sexual politics, men, feminism and politics', in V.J. Seidler (ed.) *The Achilles Heel Reader. Men, Sexual Politics and Socialism*, London: Routledge.

Self, W. (1993) *Cock and Bull*, London: Penguin.

Shaffir, W.B. (1991) 'Managing a convincing self-presentation: some personal reflections on entering the field', in W.B. Shaffir and R.A. Stebbins (eds) *Experiencing Fieldwork: An Inside View of Qualitative Research*, London: Sage.

Shaffir, W.B. and Stebbins, R.A. (eds) (1991) *Experiencing Fieldwork: An Inside View of Qualitative Research*, London: Sage

Sheffield Centre for HIV and Sexual Health (1993) 'Flirting fancying and boundaries, gay culture and professional practice in HIV prevention', Sheffield: Sheffield Centre for HIV and Sexual Health.

—— (1996) 'Who's cruising who? Boundary issues for gay and bisexual men involved in HIV and sexual health work', Sheffield: Sheffield Centre for HIV and Sexual Health.

Shepherd, J., Turner, G. and Weare, K. (1999) 'A new method of peer-led HIV prevention with gay and bisexual men', in P. Aggleton, G. Hart and P.M. Davies (eds) *Families and Communities Responding to AIDS*, London: UCL Press.

Sheppard, D.L. (1989) 'Organizations, power and sexuality: the image and self-image of women managers', in J. Hearn, D.L. Sheppard, P. Tancred-Sheriff and G. Burrell (eds) *The Sexuality of Organization*, London: Sage.

Shilts, R. (1987) *And the Band Played On: People, Politics and the AIDS Crisis*, London: Penguin.

Silverman, D. (1991) 'On throwing away the ladders: rewriting the theory of organisations', paper presented to Towards a New Theory of Organisations Conference, Keele University, April 1991, London: Goldsmiths' College (mimeo).

—— (1994) *Interpreting Qualitative Data: Methods for Analysing Talk, Text and Interaction*, London: Sage.

Simpson, M. (1995) 'Unholy trinity', *Time Out*, 8–15 February, 1277: 90.

Singer, M. (1993) 'Knowledge for use: anthropology and community-centred substance abuse research', *Social Science Medicine* 37(1): 15–25.

Small, N. (1994) 'The changing context of health care in the UK: implications for HIV/AIDS services', in P. Aggleton, P. Davies and G. Hart (eds) *AIDS: Foundations For the Future*, London: Taylor and Francis.

Smith, D. (1988) *The Everyday World as Problematic: A Feminist Sociology*, Milton Keynes: Open University Press.

Snipe, A.W.R. (1995) *Sex, Priests and Power: Anatomy of a Crisis*, New York: Brunner/Mazel.

Society for the Scientific Study of Sex (1993) 'Statement of ethical guidelines', *Journal of Sex Research* May, 30(2): 192–8.

Song, M. and Parker, D. (1995) 'Cultural identity: disclosing commonality and difference in in-depth interviewing, *Sociology* 29(2): 241–57.

Stacey, M. and Price, M. (1981) *Women, Power and Politics*, London: Tavistock.

Stanley, L (1982) ' "Male needs": the problems and problems of working with gay men', in S. Friedman and E. Sarah (eds) *On the Problem of Men: Two Feminist Conferences*, London: The Women's Press.

Stow, D. (1996) *HIV and Sexual Health Outreach MWHSWM, Review of Year 1*, Luton: South Bedfordshire Community Health Care Trust.

Strauss, A. (1969) *Mirrors and Masks: The Search for Identity*, San Francisco: The Sociology Press.

Strauss, A., Fagerhaugh, S., Suczeck, B. and Wiener, C. (1985) *The Social Organization of Medical Work*, Chicago: University of Chicago Press.

Sullivan, O. (2000) 'The division of domestic labour: twenty years of change?', *Sociology* 34(3): 437–56.

Taylor, M. (1995) 'Lest we forget', *The Trust Newsletter* May, 37: 5.

Teeman, T. (1995) 'Future AIDS campaigns set to target gay men', *Pink Paper*, 8 December.

The Trend Letter (1997) '15 Major Trends for 1998', *Special Issue*, London: The Global Network.

Thomas, L. (1995) 'Vicars given sexual ten commandments', *Sunday Times* 27 August, 8922: 1.

Thompson, P. and Ackroyd, S. (1994) 'Ain't misbehavin: power and consent in organisation sexuality', paper presented to British Sociological Association Conference 1994 (mimeo).

Thud (1996) 'Cottage Pi-ous', *Thud* 9 August.

Time Out (1995) Talking hearts column, *Time Out*, October, 1311, 4–11: 158.

Times Educational Supplement (1995) 'Think before you leap into bed, members urged', *Times Educational Supplement*.

Tonkiss, F. and Passey, A. (1999) 'Trust, confidence and voluntary organisations: between values and institutions', *Sociology* 33(2): 57–274.

Torrington, J. (1994) *Swing Hammer Swing*, London: Minerva.

Torstendahl, R. (1990) 'Introduction: promotion and strategies of knowledge-based groups', in R. Torstendahl and M. Burrage (eds) *The Formation of Professions*, London: Sage.

Treichler, P.A. (1991) 'How to have theory in an epidemic: the evolution of AIDS treatment activism', in C. Penley and A. Ross (eds) *Technoculture*, Cultural Politics vol. 3, Oxford: University of Minnesota Press.

Tucker, J. (2000) 'Working relationships', *Elle* December: 292–6.

Turner, L. (2000) 'The end of the office affair', *London Evening Standard* 6 October: 30–31.

Udry, J.R. (1993) 'The politics of sex research', *Journal of Sex Research* 30(2): 103–10.

Ussher, J. (1993) 'Paradoxical practices: psychologists as scientists in the field of AIDS', in C. Squire (ed.) *Women and AIDS: Psychological Perspectives* London: Sage.

Ussher, J. (1996) 'Putting the pleasure back into sex', *New Scientist* 3 February: 41.

Vance, C. (1991) 'Anthropology rediscovers sexuality: a theoretical comment', *Social Science Medicine* 33(8): 875–84.

Van Maanen, J. (1991) 'Playing back the tape. Early days in the field', in W.B. Shaffir and R.A. Stebbins (eds) *Experiencing Fieldwork, An Inside View of Qualitative Research*, London: Sage.

Van Reyk, P. (1990) 'On the beat: a report on an outreach program of AIDS preventative education for men who have sex with men', Darlinghurst: AIDS Council of New South Wales (mimeo).

Wagenhauser, J. (1991) 'Safe sex without condoms', *Outlook* Winter: 65–70.

Wakeling (1993) 'Wounded healers: awakenings', in J. Walmsley, J. Reynolds, P. Shakespeare and R. Woolfe (eds) *Health Welfare and Practice: Reflecting on Roles and Relationships*, London: Open University Press/Sage.

Ward, P. and Jones, J. (1996) 'The phase that dare not speak its name', in K. Deverell (ed.) *Building Bridges, Linking Research and Primary HIV Prevention, Conference Report*, London: NAM Publications.

Warren, C.A.B. and Rasmussen, P.K. (1977) 'Sex and gender in field research', *Urban Life* October, 6(3): 349–69.

Watney, S. (1987) 'People's perceptions of the risk of AIDS and the role of the mass media', *Health Education Journal* 46(2): 62–5.

—— (1989) 'Taking liberties: an introduction', in E. Carter and S. Watney (eds) *Taking Liberties: AIDS and Cultural Politics*, London: Serpent's Tail.

—— (1990a) 'Practices of freedom: "Citizenship" and the politics of identity in the age of AIDS', in J. Rutherford (ed.) *Identity, Community, Culture, Difference*, London: Lawrence and Wishart.

—— (1990b) 'Safer sex as community practice', in P. Aggleton, P. Davies and G. Hart (eds) *AIDS: Individual, Cultural and Policy Dimensions*, London: Falmer.

—— (1990c) 'Putting the gay back into AIDS', *Pink Paper* 20 October, 145: 12–13.

—— (1991) 'AIDS: the second decade: risk, research and modernity', in P. Aggleton, P. Davies and G. Hart (eds) *AIDS: Responses, Interventions and Care*, London: Falmer.

—— (1994) 'A passion for friends', *Pink Paper* 15 April, 323: 11.

—— (1995a) 'Shaming and blaming', *Pink Paper* 3 November.

—— (1995b) 'Moving targets: some reflections on the origins and history of Gay Men Fighting AIDS', *F***Sheet* November, 19: 1–3.

Weatherburn, P., Davies, P.M., Hunt, A.J., Coxon, A.P.M. and McManus, T.J. (1991) 'Condom use in a large cohort of homosexually active men in England and Wales', *AIDS Care* 2(4): 319–24.

Weatherburn, P., Hunt, A.J., Hickson, F.C.I. and Davies, P.M. (1992) *The Sexual Lifestyles of Gay and Bisexual Men in England and Wales*, London: Department of Health.

Weeks, J. (1990) 'The value of difference', in J. Rutherford (ed.) *Identity, Community, Culture, Difference*, London: Lawrence and Wishart.

—— (1991) *Against Nature: Essays on History, Sexuality and Identity*, London: Rivers Oram Press.

—— (1995) *Invented Moralities: Sexual Values in an Age of Uncertainty*, Oxford: Polity.

Weeks, J., McKevitt, C., Parkinson, K., Taylor-Labourn, A. and Aggleton, P. (1994) 'The community based response to HIV and AIDS reconsidered: The "de-gaying" and "re-gaying" of AIDS', paper presented at British Sociological Association Conference 1994 (mimeo).

Weston, C. (1992) 'Sex pests found in workplaces across the board says survey', *Guardian* 1 June.

Westwood, S. (1984) *All Day Everyday. Factory and Family in the Making of Women's Lives*, London: Pluto Press.

Wheatley, M.J. (1994) *Leadership and the New Science, Learning about Organization from an Orderly Universe*, San Francisco: Berrett-Koehler.

Whinnery, S. (1993) 'Tales of unsafe sex', *F***Sheet*, November, 2: 2.

Whitehead, T. (1989) 'Government complacency', *Capital Gay*, 22 September, 411: 4.

Whyte, D. (1996) *The Heart Aroused, Poetry and the Preservation of the Soul in Corporate America*, London: Currency Doubleday.

Williams, J. (1993) 'What is a profession? Experience versus expertise', in J. Walmsley, J. Reynolds, P. Shakespeare and R. Woolfe (eds) *Health Welfare and Practice: Reflecting on Roles and Relationships*, London: Open University Press/Sage.

Williams, W. (1993) 'Being gay and doing research on homosexuality in non-Western cultures', *Journal of Sex Research* 30(2): 115–20.

Winterson, J. (1990) *Sexing the Cherry*, London: Vintage.

Witz, A. (1992) *Professions and Patriarchy*, London: Routledge.

Wright-Mills, C. (1983) *The Sociological Imagination*, London: Penguin.

Index